QUICK LOOK NURSING
HUMAN GROWTH AND DEVELOPMENT THROUGH THE LIFESPAN

QUICK LOOK NURSING

Human Growth and Development Through the Lifespan

Kathleen M. Thies, Ph.D., RN

Chair and Director of Nursing
Colby-Sawyer College
New London, New Hampshire

John F. Travers, EdD

Department of Counseling, Developmental Psychology, and Research Methods
Boston College
Boston, Massachusetts

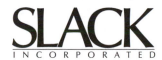

SLACK
INCORPORATED

an innovative information, education and management company
6900 Grove Road • Thorofare, NJ 08086

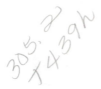

Publisher: John H. Bond
Editorial Director: Amy E. Drummond
ISBN 1-55642-506-6
Copyright © 2001 by SLACK Incorporated

The procedures and practices described in this book should be implemented in a manner consistent with the professional standards set for the circumstances that apply in each specific situation. Every effort has been made to confirm the accuracy of the information presented and to correctly relate generally accepted practices. The author, editor, and publisher cannot accept responsibility for errors or exclusions or for the outcome of the application of the material presented herein. There is no expressed or implied warranty of this book or information imparted by it.

Care has been taken to ensure that drug selection and dosages are in accordance with currently accepted/ recommended practice. Due to continuing research, changes in government policy and regulations, and various effects of drug reactions and interactions, it is recommended that the reader review all materials and literature provided for each drug, especially those that are new or not frequently used.

Any review or mention of specific companies or products is not intended as an endorsement by the author or the publisher.

Published by: SLACK Incorporated
          6900 Grove Road
          Thorofare, NJ 08086 USA
          Telephone: 856-848-1000
          Fax: 856-853-5991
          World Wide Web: www.slackbooks.com

Published in the United States of America

Contact SLACK Incorporated for more information about other books in this field or about the availability of our books from distributors outside the United States.

Last digit is print number: 10 9 8 7 6 5 4 3 2 1

Contents

Preface   vii
Introduction: The Nature of Human Development   ix
Abbreviations   xi

PART I. MAJOR THEORIES AND ISSUES

Chapter 1
Freud: Psychoanalytic Theory   2
Chapter 2
Erikson: Eight Stages of the Life Cycle   4
Chapter 3
Piaget: Universal Constructivist Perspective   6
Chapter 4
Vygotsky: Culture and Development   8
Chapter 5
Bronfenbrenner: Ecology of Human
Development   10
Chapter 6
Maslow: Humanistic Perspective on
Development   12
Chapter 7
Pavlov, Skinner, and Bandura: Learning
Perspective on Development   14
Chapter 8
A Cultural Perspective on Development   16
Chapter 9
Gender Differences   18
Chapter 10
A Social Class Perspective on Development   20

Part I: Questions   22
Part I: Answers and Explanations   24

PART II. PRENATAL DEVELOPMENT

Chapter 11
Genes, Chromosomes, and DNA   28
Chapter 12
Fertilization in Utero   30
Chapter 13
Conception to Birth   32
Chapter 14
Infertility   34
Chapter 15
Assisted Reproductive Techniques   36
Chapter 16
The Human Genome Project   38
Chapter 17
Genetic Defects   40

Chapter 18
Chromosomal Abnormalities   42
Chapter 19
Influences on Prenatal Development   44
Chapter 20
Hazards of Prematurity—Part A   46
Chapter 21
Hazards of Prematurity—Part B   48
Chapter 22
Adoption   50

Part II: Questions   52
Part II: Answers and Explanations   54

PART III. INFANCY

Chapter 23
Neonatal Assessment   58
Chapter 24
Reflexes   60
Chapter 25
Growth and Development I   62
Chapter 26
Growth and Development II   64
Chapter 27
Brain Development   66
Chapter 28
Cognitive Development   68
Chapter 29
Language Development   70
Chapter 30
First Relationships   72
Chapter 31
Attachment   74
Chapter 32
Emotional Development   76

Part III: Questions   78
Part III: Answers and Explanations   80

PART IV. EARLY CHILDHOOD

Chapter 33
Growth and Motor Development   84
Chapter 34
Cognitive Development—Part A   86
Chapter 35
Cognitive Development—Part B   88
Chapter 36
Early Childhood Education   90

Chapter 37
Language Development — 92
Chapter 38
Role of the Family — 94
Chapter 39
Homeless Children — 96
Chapter 40
Divorce — 98
Chapter 41
Day Care — 100
Chapter 42
Development of Self — 102
Chapter 43
Gender Development—Part A — 104
Chapter 44
Gender Development—Part B — 106
Chapter 45
Play Behavior — 108

Part IV: Questions — 110
Part IV: Answers and Explanations — 112

PART V. MIDDLE CHILDHOOD

Chapter 46
Growth and Development — 116
Chapter 47
Cognitive Development — 118
Chapter 48
Intelligence — 120
Chapter 49
Problem Solving — 122
Chapter 50
Moral Development — 124
Chapter 51
Language Development — 126
Chapter 52
Peers and Social Development — 128
Chapter 53
Schools and Learning — 130
Chapter 54
Encouraging Creativity in Children — 132
Chapter 55
Resilience in Childhood — 134
Chapter 56
Exceptional Children — 136

Part V: Questions — 138
Part V: Answers and Explanations — 140

PART VI. ADOLESCENCE

Chapter 57
Puberty — 144

Chapter 58
Health — 146
Chapter 59
Sexuality — 148
Chapter 60
Cognitive Development — 150
Chapter 61
Adolescent Thought — 152
Chapter 62
Peer Relationships — 154
Chapter 63
The Search for Identity — 156
Chapter 64
Motivating Adolescents — 158
Chapter 65
Delinquency — 160
Chapter 66
Mental Health Problems — 162

Part VI: Questions — 164
Part VI: Answers and Explanations — 165

PART VII. ADULTHOOD

Chapter 67
Early Adulthood: Physical Health — 170
Chapter 68
Early Adulthood: Cognitive Development — 172
Chapter 69
Early Adulthood: Psychosocial Development — 174
Chapter 70
Middle Adulthood: Physical Health — 176
Chapter 71
Middle Adulthood: Cognitive Development — 178
Chapter 72
Middle Adulthood: Psychosocial Development — 180
Chapter 73
Later Adulthood: Physical Health — 182
Chapter 74
Later Adulthood: Cognition — 184
Chapter 75
Later Adulthood: Psychosocial
Development—Part A — 186
Chapter 76
Later Adulthood: Psychosocial
Development—Part B — 188

Part VI: Questions — 190
Part VI: Answers and Explanations — 191

References — 193
Figure Credits — 201
Index — 203

Preface

For nurses and physicians, insights into the peaks and valleys of human development afford unique opportunities to further their relationships with colleagues and patients. As we come to the birth of a new century, new theories, new techniques, and new views of human nature offer hope for a more penetrating understanding of the path of human development. A major task for all nursing students is to understand human development—the characteristics, problems, and needs of people of various ages—so that they can utilize their knowledge and expertise as fully as possible in bringing comfort to their patients.

K.M.T
J.F.T

The Nature of Development

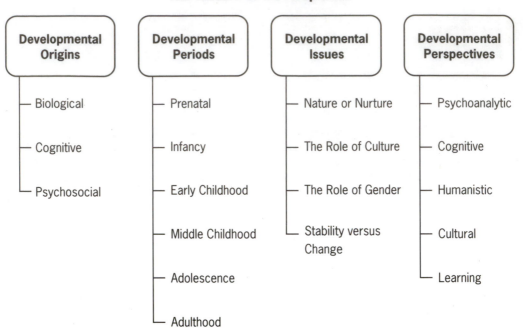

Developmental Origins
- Biological
- Cognitive
- Psychosocial

Developmental Periods
- Prenatal
- Infancy
- Early Childhood
- Middle Childhood
- Adolescence
- Adulthood

Developmental Issues
- Nature or Nurture
- The Role of Culture
- The Role of Gender
- Stability versus Change

Developmental Perspectives
- Psychoanalytic
- Cognitive
- Humanistic
- Cultural
- Learning

Introduction: The Nature of Human Development

Human development is the process that produces physical and psychosocial changes throughout the life span, from conception to death. Physical changes include obvious accomplishments such as the transformation of an apparently helpless infant into a walking, talking 2-year-old. Development also encompasses less obvious psychosocial changes such as the emergence of ever-more complex language patterns and the ability to understand obscure, even hidden, meanings. Attempting to address how these developmental changes occur leads us to search for the underlying mechanisms that explain growth and development.

Developmental Origins

Complicating the search for explanations of human development is the interaction of biological, cognitive, and psychosocial forces (see **Figure**). For example, 7-year-old children typically reverse their thinking; that is, they can explain how they arrived at an answer by retracing their steps. If you pour water from 1 bottle into a taller, thinner bottle, the level of the water will be higher. Almost all 7-year-olds, however, will tell you it is the same amount of water. When you ask them how they know, they will tell you that *they poured it back in their heads.*

These changes reflect a combination of physical forces (brain development), cognitive forces (intelligence), and psychosocial forces (environments). The interaction of these developmental influences is referred to as *biopsychosocial interactions*. (For a detailed discussion of this concept, see Dacey and Travers, 1999.) A key to understanding human development is the search for the interactions that produce development.

Developmental Periods

The human life span can be divided into segments that help to recall and integrate the main features of each period. We have divided the life span as follows:
* *Prenatal period.* Topics such as fertilization techniques, genetic discoveries (including the ongoing findings of the Human Genome Project), the developmental milestones of the prenatal months, and many of the hazards that lead to early problems are

reviewed. Our purpose is to call attention to the significant accomplishments of the months that result in an active, adaptive human being at birth.
* *Infancy (0–2 years).* This is a time when physical and psychosocial changes appear with amazing rapidity. Walking and talking are 2 observable changes, but sophisticated interactions between infants and the adults around them establish the basis of future social relationships.
* *Early childhood (2–7 years).* Growth continues at a slightly slower rate, while language and cognitive development indicate abstract ability. Peers become more important, and children acquire a good idea of who they are (their sense of self) as they steadily enlarge their circle of social relationships.
* *Middle childhood (7–12 years).* The cognitive skills that enable children to engage in ever-more abstract activities (solving problems, demonstrating creativity) emerge. As their childhood world expands, they encounter increasing and varied forms of stimulation from friends, school, and the media.
* *Adolescence.* The search for identity, coupled with physical and psychosocial changes, produces an intense preoccupation with the self.
* *Adulthood.* A range of developmental tasks arise that must be mastered if successful aging is to occur. Marriage, family, health, finances, and the inevitable problems associated with aging characterize these years.

Developmental Issues

Nature or Nurture

In the study of human development, certain themes appear with considerable regularity. One example is the issue of whether inborn tendencies (nature) or the surrounding world (nurture) exert greater influence on development. In other words, which one is more decisive for development, genes or environments? Most developmental psychologists lean toward an interplay between these two forces in shaping development: The *interaction* between genes and environment explains a person's development. Humans, using their genetic heritages, interact with their environments, not as passive recipients but as active shapers of their destinies.

The Role of Culture.

The relationship of culture to human development is critical in society, as interactions with members of different cultures occur on a daily basis. Responses to others who seem different can have a serious impact on achievement in school, success in work, and harmonious relationships. For example, patients from different cultures may well interact with nurses and physicians in a different manner. Their learning styles may vary, which can affect the way they think about medication. All of these conditions have developmental consequences.

The Role of Gender.

Gender is a powerful psychosocial factor in development. Although stereotypical thinking about males and females is slowly declining, if people are treated according to rigid role characteristics, then their potential is immediately limited. Children quickly construct social categories from the world around them, attach certain characteristics to these categories, and then label the categories. This process is positive in that it helps children to organize their world, but it may be negative if the characteristics associated with a particular category are limiting (e.g., "girls just can't do math").

Stability versus Change.

This is another issue that impacts the relationship between nurses and clients. Humans show amazing resiliency, which testifies to an ability to change. Yet resiliency has its limits, which testifies to the lingering effects of stability. Most developmental psychologists would argue for the presence of both stability and change.

Developmental Perspectives

One way of organizing developmental data into a meaningful body of knowledge is by the use of theories. A theory is an integrated set of ideas that helps one to comprehend and bring order to a mass of factual data. We urge you to select the features of each of the following theories that you believe best explain a certain aspect of development:

- *Psychoanalytic theory.* Perhaps best known because of the work of *Sigmund Freud* and *Erik Erikson,* this theory attempts to explain human development, especially personality development, as the product of unconscious forces. Erikson, while in basic agreement with Freud, placed greater emphasis on a person's environment (family, school, friends) in development.

- *Cognitive theory.* The cognitive perspective on human development has perhaps been best expressed by *Jean Piaget,* who believed that cognitive development proceeds as cognitive structures develop. The changing nature of the cognitive structures led Piaget to speculate that intellectual development comes about in a series of stages: sensorimotor, preoperational, concrete operational, and formal operational.

- *Humanistic theory. Abraham Maslow,* an adherent of the humanistic school of psychology, believed that an individual's basic needs must be satisfied if normal development is to take place. Maslow formulated a hierarchy of needs that, if satisfied, eventually would lead to a feeling of self-actualization.

- *Cultural or contextual theory.* A different interpretation of cognitive development, known as the cultural or contextual perspective, was proposed by *Lev Vygotsky.* Vygotsky believed that the clues to understanding cognitive development can be found in a person's social process (i.e., the interactions that people have with those around them). Uri Bronfenbrenner, working within the cultural-contextual framework, stressed the importance of the environment in shaping people's lives. He proposed a system analysis of development. Identifying several systems (microsystem, mesosystem, exosystem, and macrosystem), Bronfenbrenner believed that an individual's growth is influenced by an ever-expanding environmental network.

- *Learning theory.* Finally, psychologists such as *B. F. Skinner* have long argued that the best explanation of development lies in learning. Skinner, using a learning perspective, argued that development proceeds when a person's behavior is reinforced. An offshoot of Skinner's work is called the *social cognitive learning perspective.* Popularized by Albert Bandura, this perspective turned to modeling or observational learning to explain how people behave and develop as they do. In other words, by observing the behavior of others, people learn their way through life.

We develop each of these theories in greater detail in Part I, to illustrate the complexities of human development.

Introduction References

Dacey, J., Travers, J. (1999). *Human development across the lifespan (4th ed.).* New York: McGraw-Hill.

Abbreviations

A	adenine		IDDM	insulin-dependent diabetes mellitus
ADA	Americans with Disabilities Act		IDEA	Individuals with Disabilities Education Act
ADD	attention deficit disorder		IUD	intrauterine device
ADHD	attention deficit hyperactivity disorder		IVF	in vitro fertilization
AGA	appropriate for gestational age		kcal	kilocalorie
AIDS	acquired immunodeficiency syndrome		kg	kilograms
AIP	artificial insemination by partner		lb	pound
ART	assisted reproductive technology		LBW	low birth weight
BADL	bodily activities of daily living		LDL	low-density lipoprotein
BNBAS	Brazelton Neonatal Behavioral Assessment Scale		LEP	limited English proficiency
			LH	luteinizing hormone
BPD	bronchopulmonary dysplasia		mg	milligrams
C	cytosine		mL	milliliter
CF	cystic fibrosis		mRNA	messenger ribonucleic acid
cm	centimeter		NAEYC	National Association for the Education of Young Children
CMV	cytomegalovirus			
CNS	central nervous system		NICHD	National Institute of Child Health and Development
CVD	cardiovascular disease			
dL	deciliters		NIH	National Institutes of Health
DNA	deoxyribonucleic acid		NYLS	New York Longitudinal Study
DOE	Department of Energy		oz	ounce
DSM-IV	Diagnostic and Statistical Manual of Mental Disorders, 4th edition		PCBs	polychlorinated biphenyls
			PID	pelvic inflammatory disease
EDC	estimated date of confinement		PIVH	periventricular-intraventricular hemorrhage
EEG	electroencephalogram		PKU	phenylketonuria
ELSI	ethical, legal, and social issues		PNS	peripheral nervous system
ERT	estrogen replacement therapy		PTSD	posttraumatic stress disorder
ESL	English as a second language		RDS	respiratory distress syndrome
FSH	follicle-stimulating hormone		RNA	ribonucleic acid
FTT	failure to thrive		SAT	Scholastic Assessment Test
G	guanine		SES	social and economic status
g	gram		SGA	small for gestational age
GIFT	gamete intrafallopian transfer		STDs	sexually transmitted diseases
GnRH	gonadotropin-releasing hormone		T	thymidine
HGP	Human Genome Project		VLBW	very low birth weight
HIV	human immunodeficiency virus		ZIFT	zygote intrafallopian transfer
IADL	independent activities of daily living			

PART I
Major Theories and Issues

1 Freud: Psychoanalytic Theory

A Defense mechanisms

Mechanism	Explanation/Example
Rationalization	Creation of false but plausible excuses to justify behavior. Example: "Everyone else does it."
Repression	Way of keeping anxiety-producing thoughts in the unconscious. Example: "Forgetting" a troubling experience.
Projection	Attributing your thoughts, feelings, or motives to somebody else. Example: believing a co-worker for whom you have sexual feelings has made a pass at you.
Displacement	Diverting feelings that you have toward someone away from that person and toward another person or object. Example: Yelling at your spouse when you are angry at your boss.
Reaction formation	Behaving in a way that is exactly opposite the way you feel. Example: Crusading against pornography when you secretly enjoy it.
Regression	Reverting to immature behavior. Example: Adult temper tantrums.
Identification	Aligning yourself with a person or group that you admire as a way to form a positive self-identity. Example: Joining a sorority.

B Stages of psychosexual development

Stage	Age	Focus of Sexual Urges
Oral	First year of life	The mouth, e.g., sucking, biting
Anal	Toddler	Controlling biological urges, e.g., bowel movements.
Phallic	3–5 yr	Genital self-pleasure; the Oedipus complex
Latency	5 yr–puberty	Suppressing urges
Genital	Puberty	Peers of opposite sex

C Key points

Pleasure principle: we act to gratify instinctual desires and avoid pain.

Unconscious forces govern our behavior.

Childhood experiences have a strong influence on adult personality.

Personality is shaped by how we control our sexual urges.

Born in 1856, Sigmund Freud was raised in Vienna, the son of a Jewish merchant. After completing medical school in 1886, Freud began practicing neurology, specializing in hysteria. Concluding its origins were sexual in nature, he developed psychoanalytic techniques to encourage patients to recall past experiences. When female patients reported prepubertal sexual encounters with their fathers, Freud struggled with deciding whether these encounters were fantasies or actual events. He underwent self-analysis and his theory of psychosexual development evolved from this process.

Freud indulged in cocaine to relieve depression, but addiction to nicotine caused his death from cancer of the mouth. In 1938, he left Vienna in poor health to seek refuge from the Nazis, who had destroyed his Vienna Psychoanalytic Society. He died in London in 1939.

Structure of Personality

Freud divided personality into 3 components: id, ego, and superego. His concept of the *id* was influenced by Darwin, the id is the seat of instinctual drives, especially sex, food, and aggression. Operating on the pleasure principle, the id seeks immediate gratification and wants to avoid physical and psychic pain. The id engages in primary process thinking, which is illogical and indulges in fantasy.

The id's self-serving drive for pleasure conflicts with society's norms for acceptable behavior. The *ego* emerges from this conflict, and works to keep the id out of trouble. It balances the id's drives with society's expectations by making decisions based on the reality principle, delaying immediate gratification until socially appropriate means for meeting instinctual drives can be found. The ego engages in secondary process thinking, which is realistic, and tries to solve problems.

The *superego* is the moral component of the personality. Emerging around ages 3–5 years, the superego represents an internalization of social standards for good and bad behavior. It is the individual's way of policing his or her own behavior. When the superego becomes too demanding, the individual feels excessive guilt for failing to meet moral perfection. In the absence of a superego, the individual feels no remorse.

Levels of Awareness and Dreams

Freud identified 3 levels of awareness: conscious, preconscious, and unconscious. The conscious consists of awareness of the present. The preconscious lies just below the surface, housing material that the individual knows but is not thinking about right now. The unconscious contains memories, thoughts, and desires of which the individual is not aware but which may have a profound influence on behavior, such as hostile feelings toward a loved one. The id rests entirely in the unconscious. In his 1899 book, *The Interpretation of Dreams*, Freud said the "royal road" to the unconscious is dreams.

Conflict and Defense Mechanisms

Freud believed that the internal battles between the id, ego, and superego create conflict in the personality.

The drives for sex and aggression are particularly conflicted because they are subject to ambiguous social norms, also known as mixed messages, and thus are more likely to be unfulfilled. Unconscious internal battles produce anxiety, which can slip into consciousness and cause distress. Defense mechanisms (see **Part A**), protect the ego from unpleasant feelings, especially anxiety and guilt. These include rationalization, repression, projection, displacement, reaction formation, regression, and identification.

Stages of Psychosexual Development

Freud used the term "sexual" broadly, meaning an innate drive for physical pleasures. Freud proposed that children's control over these urges progresses through 5 psychosexual stages (see **Part B**). The failure to progress is referred to as *fixation*.

During the *oral stage* in the first year of life, the main source of pleasure is the mouth, such as sucking and biting. Adult oral fixations include smoking and eating.

The *anal stage* focuses on the toddler's pleasure in controlling bowel movements. Toilet training represents society's first effort to control the child's self-serving physical drives, causing conflict between child and caretakers. Adult anal fixations involve anxiety about being punished for not performing.

The *phallic stage* occurs between the third and fifth years. Boys find pleasure in self-stimulation, and compete with their fathers for the affection of their mothers. Freud thought that girls envied boys' ability for self-pleasure, and blamed their mothers for their lack of a penis. Girls compensate for this "deficiency" by forming an attachment to their fathers. The Oedipus complex refers to sexual desires for the parent of the opposite sex accompanied by hostility toward the parent of the same sex. Freud believed that the resolution of this conflict is essential for healthy gender identification with the parent of the same sex. The conflict coincides with the emergence of the superego.

During the *latency stage*, from age 5 through puberty, sexual urges become suppressed as they form social relationships beyond the family, especially with peers.

The *genital stage* begins with puberty. During adolescence, sexual urges can be appropriately directed toward peers of the opposite sex.

Psychoanalysis

The goal of psychoanalysis is to bring into awareness unconscious conflicts, motives, and defenses so that they can be resolved. Free association is the spontaneous expression of thoughts and feelings. Interpretation involves the analyst's attempt to explain the meaning of the client's experience, including symbolism in dreams. The analyst uses the client's resistance to interpretation to further understand underlying conflicts. Transference occurs when clients relate to their analysts in ways that are similar to other significant relationships in their lives. Countertransference refers to the analyst's response to the client.

2 Erikson: Eight Stages of the Life Cycle

A Stages of life cycle

Developmental Crisis	Period	Developmental Struggle
Trust vs mistrust	Infancy	I can trust others and thus myself, vs I can't trust, my needs are unworthy.
Autonomy vs shame and doubt	Toddler	"I am", and "I can", and that's good, vs "I can't", and I am bad.
Initiative vs guilt	Preschool	I can control my busyness, vs what I do is bad.
Industry vs inferiority	School-aged	I can make friends and do things well, vs nobody likes me and I'm stupid.
Identity formation vs identity diffusion	Adolescence	I am in tune with myself, vs I am confused, a nobody.
Intimacy vs isolation	Young adult	I share who I am with special others, vs I am alone and I have nothing to share.
Generativity vs self-absorption	Adulthood	I am making a contribution, vs it only matters if it matters to me.
Ego integrity vs disgust and despair	Senescence	This was my life and I am okay with it, vs I am filled with regret, I failed.

B Key points

The social environment influences personality development throughout life.

Individuals go through 8 normative developmental cycles.

In each crisis, the individual struggles with a developmental task.

The resolution of each crisis prepares the individual, or not, for the next one.

Earlier developmental crises can be reworked and resolved later in life.

Coined the term *identity crisis* in reference to adolescents.

Erik Homburger Erikson was born in Germany in 1902 to Danish parents. He studied child analysis at the Vienna Psychoanalytic Institute with Anna Freud, and he emigrated to the United States in 1933. He developed affiliations with Harvard, Yale, and with the University of California at Berkeley, establishing Child Guidance Clinics for the treatment of childhood psychological disturbances. Erikson and his wife Joan presented the 8 stages of the human life cycle at a White House Conference in 1950, the same year *Childhood and Society* was published. He wrote *Identity: Youth and Crisis* in 1968, a time of great upheaval among American youth. He died in Cambridge, Massachusetts, in 1994.

Theory of Psychosocial Development

While Freud emphasized internal psychosexual conflict in personality development, Erikson recognized that the social environment plays a significant role in shaping a child's sense of self. Erikson's theory of psychosocial development is based on the premise that humans interact with an ever-widening circle of people, beginning with mother and ending with mankind. Each of the 8 stages is marked by a normative developmental crisis that is resolved on a continuum between opposing positive and negative outcomes (see **Part A**). Personality is formed as a result of the resolution of these crises, leaving people with strengths and weaknesses. The mature personality represents the integration of earlier stages of development, their crises, and resolutions, into later stages.

Unlike Freud, who was pessimistic about humans' ability to overcome an unfortunate early childhood, Erikson believed that humans rework earlier crises later in life. Reworking can be growth enhancing when the overall balance of the personality is more positive than negative. If earlier crises were poorly resolved, revisiting them can be disruptive, especially when doing so coincides with accidental life crises, such as illness or death.

The 8 Stages of the Life Cycle

- **Trust versus mistrust.** Infants cannot meet their own needs for food, warmth, and comfort. When they can count others, usually their mother, to meet these needs, they feel worthy of care and develop a sense of trust in "self" and in "other." Because an attentive mother cannot meet all needs at all times, even a positive resolution includes a healthy degree of mistrust. Consistently poor caregiving leaves a child with a sense of unworthiness that can negatively influence self-identity and relationships throughout life.
- **Autonomy versus shame and doubt.** Like Freud, Erikson realized that children's ability to control their body functions poses a major developmental crisis. While toddlers attach value to exerting autonomous will, caregivers disapprove of uncivilized behaviors. In a positive resolution, toddlers gain a sense of self-

pride and autonomy when adults guide them to learn approved behavior: "I am good." Even healthy toddlers experience some shame. The more they experience disapproval without guidance, the deeper their shame and the more they doubt their own will: "I am bad."

- **Initiative versus guilt.** Preschoolers who like to do things can do the wrong thing. Like Freud, Erikson saw this stage as the birth of a conscience. A little guilt helps children keep their initiative within bounds. However, children who are overburdened by unrealistic expectations for good behavior can only fail, and believe they do bad things, stifling their natural inquisitiveness.
- **Industry versus inferiority.** During the latency period, children channel their energy into developing friendships and becoming good at things, such as academics and sports. They enjoy being productive and learn from failure. Children who do not experience themselves as competent socially, physically, or intellectually develop a sense of inadequacy and inferiority.
- **Identity formation versus identity diffusion.** Identity formation in adolescence is a cornerstone of his theory. The developmental task is to integrate childhood identifications with new biological urges, assumption of social roles, and recognition of one's abilities and limitations. During the psychological moratorium adolescents try on different identities, values, and social roles. Failure to form an identity may result in identity diffusion, of feeling like a nobody, with no sense of direction or commitment to a set of values. Identity foreclosure occurs when adolescents assume a preordained role without question.
- **Intimacy versus isolation.** Once young people are secure in their identity, they can establish intimate relationships with friends, and a loving sexual relationship. Fear of losing one's identity in a relationship can lead youth to avoid commitments, causing isolation and loneliness.
- **Generativity versus self-absorption.** Generative adults are productive members of society, guiding the younger generation, caring for elders, and contributing their talents for the betterment of all. Self-absorbed adults do not look beyond their own needs, become stagnant emotionally, and are without a core set of values.
- **Integrity versus disgust.** Individuals whose resolution of developmental crises have been relatively positive reach old age with a sense of ego integrity, and accept responsibility for what life is and was—good, bad, or indifferent. Individuals who have been emotionally isolated, self-absorbed, and without a secure identity end life in despair and regret. However, Erikson felt that it is never too late to positively reintegrate the personality, to learn life's lessons, and to mature.

3 Piaget: Universal Constructivist Perspective

A Characteristics of the 4 stages of development

Sensorimotor Period (Newborn to 24 Months)
- Divided into 6 substages.
- Begins with reflexive behavior, ends with symbolic thought (language).

Four major accomplishments:
- Object permanence: an object or a person continues to exist even when out of sight.
- Spatial relationships: in/out, up/down, gravity.
- Causality: cause and effect; e.g., push the right button, Mickey Mouse pops up.
- Time: before and after; e.g., put on clean pajamas *after* a bath.

Preoperational Period (Ages 2–7)
- Animistic thinking: attributing life to inanimate objects; e.g., dolls have feelings.
- Egocentric thinking: world is created and organized around one's self.
- Associationistic thinking: things that happen at the same time cause each other.
- Perceptually bound: pay attention to what appears to be obvious without regard to the
    constraints of physics; e.g., Santa can be in 2 malls at once.
- Centration: attend to one piece of information at a time; e.g., only see that a glass is tall
    and ignore that it is also wide.

Period of Concrete Operations (Ages 7–11)
- Logical reasoning can be done mentally using rules for operation.
- Ability to reverse sequences mentally; e.g., if 3+2=5, then 5-2=3.
- Ability to decenter when solving problems: weigh multiple pieces of information at a time;
    e.g., how much juice there is depends on both the height and width of the container.
- Perceive the underlying reality (physics); e.g., Santa cannot exist in 2 malls at once.
- Focus on the immediate, not future oriented.
- Classify objects based on at least 2 properties; e.g., sort baseball cards by team and position.

Period of Formal Operations (Adolescence)
- Abstract thinking: representing reality using symbols that can be manipulated mentally;
    e.g., symbolism in Bible stories, *x* in algebraic equations.
- Logical thinking more systematic: scientific method.
- Metacognition: thinking about thinking.
- Hypothetical/propositional reasoning: able to think "What if?", playing with different scenarios
    mentally, appreciate rules of logic.
- Future oriented.

B Key points

- Child constructs reality by interacting with environment.
- Schemata are building blocks of cognitive structures.
- Cognitive structures become more complex operations.
- Development occurs over 4 stages.
- Adaptation involves assimilation and accommodation.
- Assimilation is when we incorporate our experience into existing structures or schemata.
- Accommodation is when we modify structures to meet environmental demands.

Jean Piaget (1896–1980) spent most of his life in his native Switzerland and in France. After finishing his PhD in biology, he studied experimental psychology. In 1920, while standardizing a French version of an English intelligence test for Alfred Binet, he became fascinated by children's wrong answers. Children of the same age seemed to reason incorrectly in the same way. He suspected this was a function of intellectual maturation, rather than quantity of knowledge. His research on children's intellectual development was guided by genetic epistemology, the study of the natural unfolding of maturational processes in organisms. For example, as an apple seed matures, it does not become more seed. It changes qualitatively, into a seedling, a sapling, and then a mature tree. Similarly, Piaget saw predictable qualitative differences in how children think about things at different ages.

Piaget wrote more than 50 books on a variety of topics, including intellectual, perceptual, and moral development in children. His basic theory is presented here in brief. While there have been many challenges to and subsequent revisions of Piaget's theory, his work continues to be a major influence in the field of child development.

Universal Constructivist Theory

The term *universal constructivist* implies that all humans construct their understanding of the world in predictable ways. Piaget believed humans have a dual heredity: their physical bodies and the entire natural world. Humans are not passive organisms, but take an active role in their own development by acting on the physical environment. Piaget believed that mental life in infancy begins with motor activity. The infant who swings an arm and grasps a toy is learning about controlling the body, the nature of objects, and the relationship between body and objects. The key concepts in Piaget's constructivist theory include mental structures, organization, and adaptation.

Mental Structures

Mental structures, called cognitive structures, begin with reflexes in infancy and evolve into schemata and more complex structures called operations. For example, infants have an innate grasping reflex that causes them to wrap their fingers around an object placed in their palms. They come to control this tendency as their nervous system matures. They begin to understand how they must grasp objects of various shapes and sizes. Their schemata for grasping a teething ring will be different from their schemata for grasping a block.

Multiple schemata are organized into structures that become increasingly efficient. For example, between infancy and age 2, mental structures are organized around children's sensory and motor interactions with the environment. Piaget referred to this as the sensori-motor period (see **Part A**), the first of 4 stages of development. The infant matures from grasping blocks to throwing them to banging them together and then stacking 2 blocks.

As children mature, higher-order structures called operations develop. These are the hallmarks of the last 3 of the 4 stages of development; the cognitive stages: preoperational, concrete operational, and formal operations (see **Part A**). Operations are mental actions, allowing children to interact with the environment using their minds and not just their bodies. Piaget proposed these stages form an invariant sequence, meaning that children cannot develop formal operations until they have first developed concrete operations.

Organization

Piaget believed humans have a natural and innate tendency to organize their relationship with the environment. Just as the sapling becomes part of the tree, emerging schemata are integrated into existing ones, causing a reorganization of the whole structure. Each reorganization is of a higher order, reflecting greater coordination and complexity with cognitive maturity. Stacking 2 blocks evolves into building block cities and eventually an appreciation for the physics of architecture. Stages of development refer to predictable changes in the organization of human experience of the natural world. People organize activity lawfully, constructing a reality that makes sense at the time.

Adaptation

Humans form cognitive structures for the purposes of adapting to the environment. To Piaget, the definition of intelligence *is* adaptation, that is, an ability to effectively negotiate environmental demands. Adaptation consists of the dual processes of assimilation and accommodation. When people assimilate, they incorporate an experience into existing schemata and structures. When they cannot fit an experience into existing schemata or structures, they must accommodate, that is, modify their way of thinking to fit the experience. Accommodation can be a lot of mental work, hence, the famous line "assimilate if you can, accommodate if you must" (see **Part B**).

Let's take math as an example. A first-grade student can add 3 + 2 on paper, but adding 9 + 2 requires carrying a 1 into the next column. This is a newer variation on addition. Piaget believed there are natural limits to building structures through accommodation. That is, cognitive development is constrained by biological maturation. The typical first grader cannot yet modify the cognitive structures to accommodate multiplication and division, much less algebra. But the student of algebra can still add 3 + 2, because earlier schemata for addition have been integrated into more sophisticated mental structures.

4 Vygotsky: Culture and Development

A Vygotsky's basic concepts

Perspective: child's cognitive development proceeds by social interactions.

Basic psychological mechanism: social interactions.

Role of language: moves from external to inner speech; becomes a major influence in cognitive development.

Learning: biological processes plus social interactions produce learning.

Problem solving: speech guides planful behavior; aided by social interactions.

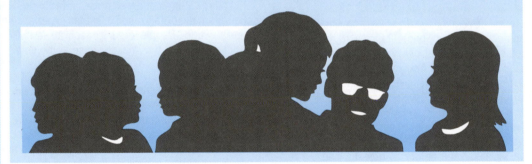

B The zone of proximal development

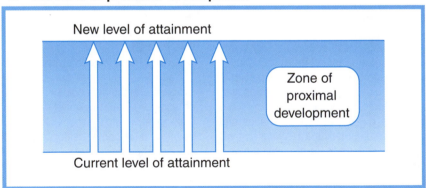

New level of attainment

Zone of proximal development

Current level of attainment

Lev Vygotsky, a Russian psychologist, has exerted a powerful influence on current developmental psychology. A theorist who thought deeply about the role of culture in development, Vygotsky was born in Russia in 1896. During his studies, he came to believe that social and cultural processes are critical for healthy growth. His career was abruptly terminated by an early death from tuberculosis in 1934, but his work is more popular now than it was when he died.

Vygotsky believed that his ideas about development were truly unique (**Part A**). He argued that development proceeds from the intersection of 2 paths: elementary processes that are basically biological, and higher psychological processes that are essentially sociocultural. For example, brain development provides the physiological basis for the appearance of external or egocentric speech, which gradually becomes the inner speech children use to guide their behavior.

The Interaction of Developmental Mechanisms

Vygotsky thought that elementary biological processes are transformed into higher psychological functioning by developmental processes. Language is a good example of what he meant. Babies make various sounds as they begin their language development (e.g., crying, cooing, babbling), all of which are accompanied by physical movement. Next, children point at objects (e.g., ball, cup, milk) and adults tell them the name. After children begin to speak their first words, they start to string words together, talk aloud, and finally, restrict speech much the way adults do.

Language and Development

Vygotsky believed that language plays a major role in development. For example, by crying, cooing, and babbling, infants immediately begin to interact with the environment and later commence to label the objects around them. When children are about 3 years old, they demonstrate egocentric speech, in which they carry on conversations whether anyone is listening or not. Gradually speech becomes internalized and begins to help them plan and guide their behavior. Vygotsky gave the example of a 4-year-old child trying to get a piece of candy from a cupboard. Initially, egocentric speech guides her behavior. Standing on a stool and searching for the candy, she says aloud, "Is that the candy?" "No, I can't get it." "I need a stick." "I can move it now." She brushes the candy to the edge of the shelf. "I can get it now. The stick worked."

The Social Origin of Mind

To understand cognitive development, Vygotsky argued that any function in a child's cultural development appears twice, on 2 planes: first, in an *interpsychological category* (social exchanges with others), and second, within the child as an *intrapsychological category* (using inner speech to guide behavior). He further argued that all higher functions (memory, thinking, problem solving) begin as relations between individuals.

Vygotsky used *internalization* to explain how external activity becomes internal activity. First, an external behavior (such as egocentric speech) is changed and begins to occur internally. Next, an interpersonal process (egocentric speech) is transformed into an intrapersonal process (inner speech). The more that children use inner speech to guide their actions, the more competent they become. Remember, however, that all mental activity results from interacting with others, which is what Vygotsky meant by the social origins of mind.

The Zone of Proximal Development

Vygotsky defined the zone of proximal development as the distance between a person's actual developmental level and the higher level of potential development. The zone of proximal development is the difference between what people can do independently and what they can do with help (**Part B**).

As an example, let's say you find yourself working with a diabetic patient who hates to exercise and whose diet leaves much to be desired. You have discovered that her eating habits are terrible: too much coffee, too many sweets, and irregular meals. She has complained frequently about "feeling tired all the time." You realize that her recovery could be slow and fatiguing if she remains on the same diet. So you work with her on improving her eating habits before she leaves. You stress the importance of regular exercise. In other words, you have guided her through Vygotsky's zone of proximal development, from what she can do on her own to what she can do with help.

Progress through the zone of proximal development depends on a person's development and intellectual possibilities. In other words, one's physical abilities (in the example, your patient's recovery level) and mental abilities (your patient's cognitive capacity to understand the value of your suggestions) will determine the extent of her recovery.

Implications for Health Care Providers

Keep in mind several key functions that lead to successful scaffolding. You must capture the interest of your patients if they are to remain focused. Keep your suggestions simple; don't make the steps to reach the goal too complicated. In the example of the patient with the poor eating habits, don't overload her with nutritional information and readings, but remind her of the good that can come from these ideas compared to the way she has been feeling. Don't hesitate to use models, selecting individuals whom the patient admires, to illustrate how the patient can maintain good health (e.g., use magazine articles or pictures).

5 Bronfenbrenner: Ecology of Human Development

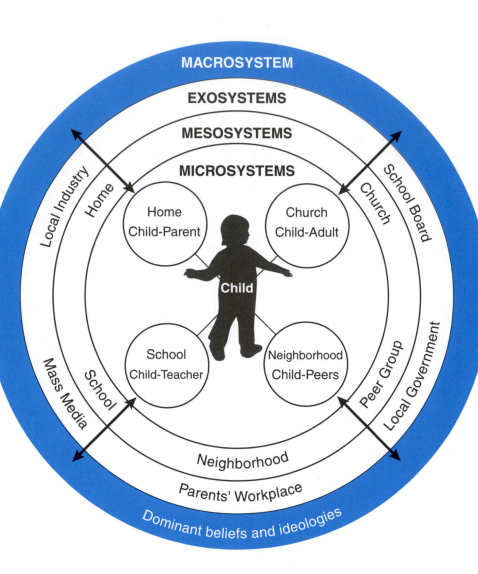

MACROSYSTEM

EXOSYSTEMS

MESOSYSTEMS

MICROSYSTEMS

Local Industry

Home

Home
Child-Parent

Church
Child-Adult

Church

School Board

Child

School
Child-Teacher

Neighborhood
Child-Peers

Mass Media

School

Peer Group

Local Government

Neighborhood

Parents' Workplace

Dominant beliefs and ideologies

Urie Bronfenbrenner, born in Russia in 1917, is a psychologist who has been a professor at Cornell University since 1948. Through his work as president of a national task force on early childhood (1966–67), he came to appreciate the multiple influences on children's school performance. In his 1979 book, *The Ecology of Human Development*, he proposed that the culture at large plays a role in children's development through the transmission of beliefs about how children should be raised and how families should function in society. He borrowed the concepts of "ecology" and "ecosystems" from the natural sciences.

Human ecology is the study of the complex interrelationships between humans and their social environments. Using his model of human ecology, he examined the impact of a variety of social and economic factors on children's development.

The Model of Human Ecology

Bronfenbrenner envisioned his model of human ecology as a "nested arrangement of concentric structures, each contained within the next" (1979, p. 22), as shown in the **Figure**. Each of the concentric structures represents a level of context in which development occurs. There are reciprocal interactions between the levels. Children impact their environments and environments impact children's development. The model consists of the following:

The innermost structure in the concentric arrangement is the *child*. Bronfenbrenner recognized that children bring to their environments their own biological makeup. For example, being male or female influences how a child is perceived by others, which in turn influences the child's behavior. Temperament, especially activity level, appears to be an inborn trait. Some children rush to the top of the jungle gym, while others quietly dig in the sand. These children impact their parents in different ways, depending on the expectations of the parents. Parents who wanted a quiet girl may be exasperated by a highly active boy, who gets the message that he is not valued, which in turn shapes the nature of his relationship with his parents.

Working outward, the next level in the concentric structures is the *microsystem*. Microsystems are the immediate social context of a child's life, the people with whom a child interacts on a regular basis. Included are parents and siblings, teachers and classmates, playmates from the neighborhood, baby-sitters, and people from church. The highly active boy may be a favorite among playmates, and the man next door loves to have him tag along when he goes to the park, but the boy drives the teenage baby-sitter crazy.

The microsystems are embedded in the *mesosystem*. This level contains community groups such as the school, neighborhood, and church or other social organizations. A coach at school might recognize the athletic prowess of the highly active boy. If the boy cannot play outside because the neighborhood is unsafe or there is no coach at school, he may channel his high energy into activities that are detrimental to the community in which he lives.

Children may not be present in the *ecosystem*, but these institutions, such as local governments, businesses, services, and media, influence children's development. A school board cuts funding for sports programs when the town cannot raise the revenue. The town struggles financially when large companies move away, taking parents' jobs and the town's tax base with them. The television station continues to cover and to glorify sports to children who can no longer participate in them. Children have an influence on these institutions as well. Teens with nothing to do can be a problem for local police.

The *macrosystem* represents the dominant beliefs and ideologies in the culture. The media cover sports because they profit financially in a capitalist society. Beliefs about children influence child-rearing practices and government policies. The cultural value placed on the primacy of the biological family has resulted in children spending years in foster homes, awaiting a reunification with unfit parents that may never come. Children also influence the macrosystem. The baby-boom generation, born between 1945 and 1960, won the right to vote at age 18 by arguing that if you can be drafted, you should be able to vote for the people drafting you.

Implications for Health Care Providers

The model of the ecology of human development is responsible for our recognition of the complex impact of social and economic status (SES) of families and communities on children. SES is more than just money. It is a marker for parental education and employment and the cohesiveness of social networks. The better educated the parents, the better off the children. Educated parents work. Working parents have organizational skills and a work ethic. They introduce their children to activities that build physical, social, and academic skills. Through these activities, children develop a sense of competence and their families become part of a network of other families in the community.

Children and families of higher SES have better access to health care and to good nutrition. Children of lower SES have difficulty getting good care, have poor diets, and engage in fewer preventative efforts. As a result, the poor have a higher incidence of chronic illness (or the chronically ill have a higher incidence of being poor because it's harder for them to stay employed).

Maslow: Humanistic Perspective on Development

A The humanistic perspective on development

Need for self-actualization

Esteem needs

Love and belongingness needs

Safety needs

Physiological needs

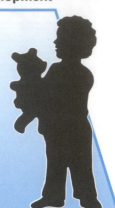

B Characteristics of self-actualized individuals

Self-actualized people

- Don't delude themselves
- Exercise sound judgment
- Accept themselves and others
- Combine spontaneity and privacy
- Meet problems and search for solutions
- Display independence and creativity

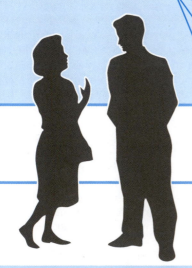

Abraham Maslow has long been associated with humanistic psychology, so called because of its focus on the fully human person. The great value of Maslow's work lies in its emphasis on psychologically healthy people. He believed that we have much to learn from people possessing an optimistic, positive outlook.

Maslow's Basic Ideas

To understand Maslow's ideas, 2 principles should be remembered: (1) Maslow was interested in studying the positive, healthy personality. (2) When peoples' basic needs are satisfied, they have the energy and drive to seek higher goals. With these as his guidelines, Maslow identified a hierarchy of needs (see **Figure**) that must be satisfied before people can move toward higher levels of thought, creativity, and self-fulfillment.

Of the basic needs Maslow identified—physiological, safety, love and belongingness, esteem, and self-actualization—the first 4 are often called *deficiency needs*. Even if these needs are satisfied, people will experience feelings of discontent or restlessness unless they are doing what they believe they should be doing. As Maslow (1987, p. 22) noted, what people can be, they must be, which leads them to attempt to satisfy *growth needs*, that is, those self-actualization needs for truth, beauty, justice, and so on.

The Hierarchy of Needs

Initially, the lower, more basic needs must be satisfied. Thus, satisfaction proceeds from bottom to top, and once these preeminent needs are satisfied, the search for self-actualization commences.

- **Physiological needs.** Maslow's premise about the physiological was simple: A hungry or thirsty person searches for food and water more keenly than for anything else. Unsatisfied physiological needs come to dominate a person's life; everything is subordinated to efforts to satisfy them. A good example of the power of this need is a patient experiencing severe pain. Nothing matters other than the need for relief from pain.
- **Safety needs.** People need to feel physically secure from threats to their lives. When this need is unmet, any concern about higher needs is lost. For example, recently a rash of tornadoes struck southern areas of the United States. Many of the individuals interviewed were not worried about financial losses, but instead expressed their thanks that they were still alive.

  People should also be free from feelings of anxiety and fear, which Maslow believed was reflected in their preferences for familiar surroundings, safe jobs, and old friends. Extreme feelings of insecurity about an illness or unwarranted fear about hospitalization can often retard a patient's recovery and signal a need for constant reassurance.

- **Love and belongingness needs.** Once physiological and safety needs are met, people can turn to giving and receiving affection, to building friendships, to establishing roots, in other words, to work at being accepted. These needs are not purely a drive for sexual satisfaction but include the notion that love involves both giving and receiving.
- **Esteem needs.** Esteem needs refer to what others think of us, as well as our opinion of ourselves. Maslow believed esteem needs reflect a desire for strength, achievement, mastery, and confidence. When these needs are met, people have positive feelings about themselves and a corresponding confidence in facing life's challenges. Maslow also believed people have a need for what he called "reputation" or "prestige." People want respect and esteem from others, but that respect or esteem must be deserved.
- **Self-actualization need.** If all the previous needs are satisfied, humans still experience feelings of discontent and restlessness unless they are doing what they believe they are uniquely suited to do. As Maslow stated (1987, p. 22), musicians must make music, artists must paint, and poets must write if they are to find peace with themselves.

Characteristics of Self-actualized People

From studying colleagues, friends, and historical figures such as Abraham Lincoln and Thomas Jefferson, Maslow identified several characteristics of self-actualized people (**Part B**). For example, self-actualized individuals have a very *accurate perception of reality*, an ability to judge people and situations correctly and efficiently. They *accept* themselves and others, recognizing, but not threatened by, the shortcomings of themselves and others. They display considerable *spontaneity*, while simultaneously welcoming *privacy*. They are *problem centered*, not focused on themselves, and are remarkably *independent* and *creative*. Although these are the more important positive characteristics, self-actualized people also have their imperfections; they can be silly, wasteful, or thoughtless, for example. Maslow's conclusion: Self-actualized people are real, not caricatures.

Implications for Health Care Providers

Maslow's ideas have important implications for health care providers. As mentioned already, satisfaction of a patient's needs substantially increases the chances of recovery. However, health care providers also have the obligation to consider their own needs if they are to offer the most professional help of which they are capable. Given the potentially dangerous consequences of many diseases, they must meet their safety needs. In addition, health care providers should work in a situation in which their esteem needs are recognized and accepted.

7

Pavlov, Skinner, and Bandura
Learning Perspective on Development

A The major learning theorists

Theorist	Key Points
Pavlov	Classical conditioning; control of stimuli
Skinner	Instrumental or operant conditioning; reinforcement schedules
Bandura	Social cognitive learning; observation, modeling

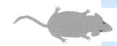

B Pavlov's classical conditioning

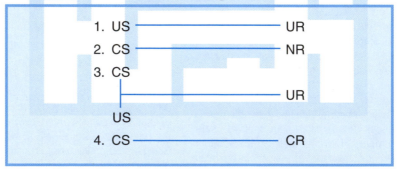

1. US ——————— UR
2. CS ——————— NR
3. CS
      |
      ——————— UR
   US
4. CS ——————— CR

Learning theorists focus on behavior; consequently, they're known as *behaviorists*. They believe that unconscious forces or unseen structures do little to further an understanding of human behavior. What is needed, they claimed, is a method that enabled observers to measure human behavior objectively and scientifically. They argued that development proceeds through learning as humans adjust to their environments. That is, the environment either rewards, punishes, or ignores us. To help you grasp the power and scope of the learning explanation of development, we consider 3 theorists: Pavlov, Skinner, and Bandura. **Part A** summarizes the key points of each of the theorists.

Pavlov's Classical Conditioning

One of the trials of childhood is receiving numerous injections. Many times you've seen pictures of children crying *before* they receive their shot, which is an excellent example of classical conditioning, discovered by the Russian physiologist Ivan Pavlov (1849–1936). Children make a response (crying) to a stimulus (the injection). On later occasions, they make a response (cry) at the sight of the stimulus (needle), perhaps at the sight of other factors associated with the stimulus (person who gives the shot). As shown in **Part B** there are 4 steps in classical conditioning that explain what happens.

Skinner's Operant Conditioning

B. F. Skinner (1904–90) developed an explanation of learning that stressed the consequences of behavior— what happens *after* we do something is all important.

For example, imagine a 10-year-old with a sweet tooth. His father has constantly prodded him all summer to mow the lawn: Do it today; do it before I get home, or else. But his mother, with a shrewd understanding of human behavior, discovers that the local store carries ice cream bars that her son likes, but they are rather expensive. She promises him a package each week after he mows the lawn. By the end of the summer he is cutting the grass on a regular basis with no threats, coercion, or scoldings. Skillful use of reinforcement greatly increased the desired behavior.

Operant Conditioning

Reinforcement, the consequence of behavior, is the key to understanding Skinner's work. For example, praise is a powerful reinforcer for people. Immediately praising a patient's desirable responses (e.g., remembering to exercise at regular intervals) is reinforcement of a specific behavior.

As you can see, the consequences of behavior—the reinforcers—are powerful controlling forces. We can summarize Skinner's thinking by saying, *control the reinforcers, control the behavior.*

Negative reinforcers also exist. These are events (also called *aversive stimuli*, something unpleasant) *removed* after a correct response appears, which then tend to increase the desired behavior. For example, chil-dren who neglect to do their homework are kept after school, thus losing their playtime. When they do what is expected—turning in homework on time—the penalty of staying after school (aversive stimulus) is removed, and they have their playtime (reinforcement). Remember: Both positive and negative reinforcement increase behavior.

Negative reinforcement should not be confused with *punishment*, which decreases behavior. What happens when those in authority withdraw a positive reinforcer (a child cannot go to the movies) or introduce something unpleasant (slapping, scolding)? Skinner believed that these conditions establish the parameters of punishment; that is, something aversive (unpleasant) appears after a response or something positive (pleasant) disappears after a response.

Social Cognitive Learning

Albert Bandura born in 1925, believed that social cognitive learning occurs through observing others, even when the observer does not reproduce the model's responses during acquisition and therefore receives no reinforcement (Bandura et al., 1963). For Bandura, *social cognitive learning* means that the information people process from observing other people, things, and events influences the way they act. Observational learning has particular relevance since we know that people do not always do what they are told, but rather what they see others do.

In a classic study, Bandura and his colleagues studied the effects of live models, filmed human aggression, and filmed cartoon aggression on preschool children's aggressive behavior. The filmed human aggression involved adult models displaying aggression toward an inflated doll; the filmed cartoon aggression involved a cartoon character displaying the same behavior as the humans; the live models displayed the identical aggression as the others. Later, all the children exhibited significantly more aggression than did youngsters in a control group. Also, filmed models were as effective as live models in transmitting aggression.

Research (Bandura, 1997) suggests that prestigious, powerful, competent models are more readily imitated than models who lack these qualities. Age, gender, race, educational, and socioeconomic qualities seem to be particularly effective in encouraging modeling.

Implications for Health Care Providers

Skinner's work has definite implications for health care providers. For example, you should be alert to the timing of reinforcement you provide. Though it may be impossible to reinforce all desirable behaviors, when you decide that a certain behavior (e.g., remembering to take medication at specified times) is critical, reinforce it immediately. Don't let time elapse. Determine precisely what you want your patients to do and then arrange a schedule so that between visits, they make as few mistakes as possible.

8 A Cultural Perspective on Development

A

Origins of the U.S. population: 1996-2050		
	1996	**2050**
White Americans	73%	53%
Hispanic Americans	11%	25%
African Americans	13%	14%
Asian Americans	4%	8%
Native Americans	1%	1%

B

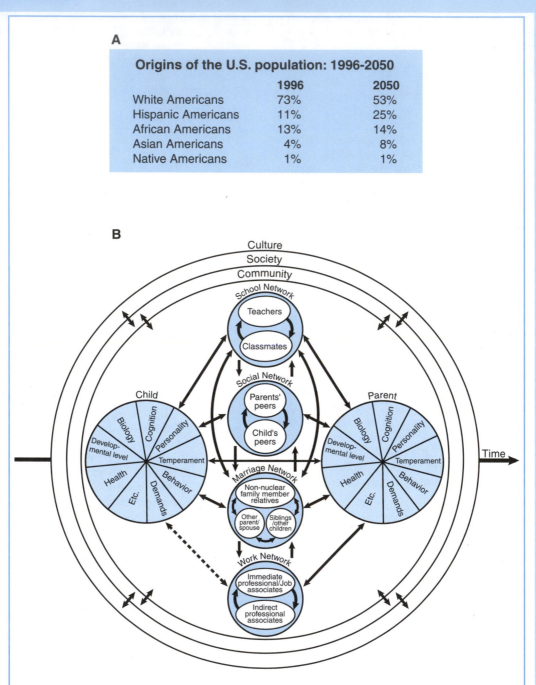

Vygotsky (discussed in Chapter 4) believed in the social origins of the human mind, recognizing the importance of culture in human development. Probably the best way to think of culture is to view it as the behavioral patterns, beliefs, attitudes, values, traditions, and other aspects of a group of people that are passed from generation to generation.

The well-known psychologist Jerome Bruner (1996) stated that culture is the framework around which humans build their minds. Human behavior emerges from unique cultural settings, which must be identified and accepted if researchers are to penetrate the secrets of development.

Part A illustrates the increasingly varied nature of the population that health care providers serve in the United States. When dealing with large numbers of patients from diverse backgrounds, remember that "different is not deficient." If your techniques and manner of interacting with others are compatible with their cultural patterns, everything improves: your relationship with your clients, their health, and your own sense of accomplishment.

Language is a good example. Today there are over 30 million Americans for whom English is not the primary language, and of them about 6 million have "limited English proficiency" (LEP). If you find yourself in a setting where most of your clients have difficulty with English, try to acquire enough conversational elements of that language to help your patients feel comfortable with you.

The Impact of Culture

Recent events in Rwanda highlight the need to recognize and capitalize on the backgrounds of your patients. Several American psychologists traveled to Rwanda to help with the massive psychological problems, particularly painful for children, caused by the heart-rending violence of the past few years. The psychologists quickly found that traditional Western therapeutic methods, such as individualized therapy, were useless.

They also discovered that urging patients to "talk it out" simply did not work. Using native songs, dances, and storytelling, which their patients found natural and comforting, proved to be much more effective. Successful programs in Africa demand programs that help restore social supports and relationships. Understanding the attitudes, customs, and behaviors—in other words, the culture—of individuals is important if you are to interact positively with them.

Developmental Contextualism

A new model was designed to illustrate how the various cultural factors interact. Called *developmental contextualism*, this model was proposed by the developmental psychologist Richard Lerner (1991) to provide a logical rationale for capitalizing on the richly diverse backgrounds of your patients. Developmental contextualism begins with the idea that all of a patient's characteristics, psychological as well as biological, interact with the environment (the context in this theory). Your patients' *context* refers to four major forces of development:

- The *physical settings* of the patients, such as the home, classroom, and workplace
- The *social influences* acting on the patients, such as their families, peers, and significant others
- The *personal characteristics* of the patients, such as physical appearance, temperament, and language fluency
- The *influence of time*, that is, the changes wrought by the experiences accumulated through the years

Part B summarizes the developmental contextual perspective.

Implications for Health Care Providers

As a health care provider, you'll want to be aware of cultural differences among your patients so that you may offer as supportive environment as possible. For example, Hispanics usually don't like to be singled out; they function more effectively when working in groups. Relationships are extremely important to them so the quality of their interactions with others is critical to them.

The same rationale applies to other groups. For example, African Americans tend to respond to the whole picture rather than parts. They tend to react better to inferential rather than deductive methods and are extremely proficient in nonverbal communication. Finally, an important point for providers to remember is that African Americans prefer to focus on people rather than things. Consequently, the manner in which you work with African-American patients is more important than merely listing things for them to do.

For example, think of a patient admitted to a hospital. Undoubtedly emotionally upset because of a disease or injury, your patient is in a physical setting that is quite different, perhaps even threatening. The patient's accustomed social setting is simply nonexistent. Looking around, the patient may see no reassuring figure. It's not too hard to imagine that personal characteristics such as speaking a different language affect the patient's emotional state. Fear and anxiety probably are on the rise, affecting everything from blood pressure to temperature. Now add to this mixture the added burden of being in a setting where the patient has had little, if any, experience.

Gender Differences

A

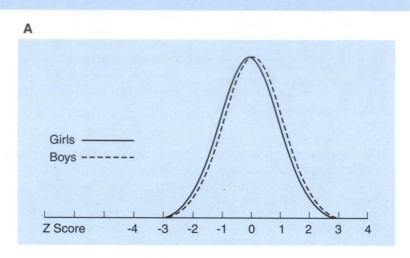

Girls ——————
Boys - - - - - -

Z Score   -4   -3   -2   -1   0   1   2   3   4

B Rod and frame test

Ignore the orientation of the frame and adjust the position of the rod so that it is vertical.

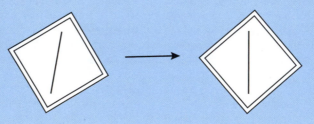

C Mental rotation

Which figure on the right is identical to the figure in the box?

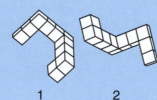
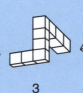
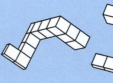

1   2   3   4   5

Gender is the most salient human characteristic. Males and females are far more similar than they are different. Nevertheless, humans are drawn to differences, and exaggerate their relevance, giving rise to stereotypes.

Research on gender differences relies on meta-analysis. Researchers use the means and standard deviations for males and females reported in many studies to calculate an "effect size." Effect size is measured in comparison to "no effect," as in "gender has no effect on aggression." Large-scale studies report gender differences in terms of variance, a statistical measure of how much of one variable (aggression) can be explained by another (gender).

When researchers look for gender differences, they examine the distribution of the scores for males and females. Most often, the distributions overlap. The area in which they do not overlap is the area of statistical difference. A small difference may be statistically significant, but of no practical importance in terms of explaining the difference, or justifying interventions to eliminate it. **Part A**, explained later, shows the overlapping normal distributions in mathematics performance for males and females.

In 1974, Maccoby and Jacklin reported 4 areas of male-female differences: verbal ability, quantitative ability, spatial ability, and aggression. Since then, meta-analyses have challenged or explained those differences.

Intellectual Performance

A popular stereotype is that girls are verbal and intuitive whereas boys are math oriented and logical. Research shows there are no gender differences in IQ. A few differences on performance on subtests have been found, but they are smaller than stereotypes propose.

Verbal Ability

Girls develop language more rapidly than boys, placing them at an advantage in reading, spelling, and writing during the early grades. Boys are more likely to have language-related problems, such as dyslexia, thus widening the perceived gap between them and girls in elementary school. The difference in performance on verbal tasks is small, with gender accounting for only 1% of the variance in meta-analyses.

By adolescence, girls still have an advantage, but the differences are more complex. Adolescent girls do better on subtests of synonyms, speech production, and word knowledge. Adolescent boys do better with analogies. The Scholastic Assessment Test (SAT) in verbal ability is heavily weighted with analogies, giving boys a slight advantage. In summary, gender differences in verbal ability are too small to be of practical importance (Lips, 1997).

Mathematical Abilities

Girls have a slight advantage over boys in arithmetic computation during the elementary school years; boys do better with problem solving. Real differences emerge during high school and college, when boys' relative skill in problem solving gives them the advantage with more complex math problems. **Part A** shows that on a meta-analysis of more than 100 samples, the distribution of male and female scores overlaps so closely that the difference is almost negligible (Friedman, 1989). When samples are drawn from the general population, no difference between males and females appears. In some studies, females outperform males. When samples are drawn from more gifted students, males outperform females.

That is, the differences found between males and females in meta-analyses may be attributed to that small subgroup of males who are unusually precocious. Even so, only 1%–5% of the variance can be explained by gender, and that gender gap has decreased in recent years as schools have paid more attention to girls' development in math (Hyde, Fenema, and Lamon, 1990). Why boys outnumber girls among the mathematically brilliant is unclear. Brain organization, social expectations, achievement motivation, and opportunity may be factors.

Spatial Abilities

Spatial perception refers to the ability to locate horizontal and vertical planes in a field with conflicting information (see **Part B**). Differences favoring males are small during childhood, becoming larger during adulthood. *Mental rotation* refers to the ability to mentally visualize a 3-dimensional object's rotation in space (see **Part C**). Males score higher than females across the life span. Women seem to have an advantage on spatial tasks that depend on perceptual speed, such as matching objects (Brannon, 1996).

Experience with spatial tasks plays a role in performance on spatial tasks (Baenninger and Newcombe, 1989). Boys who grow up building things have had more experience manipulating objects with their hands and their minds than girls. When girls participate in training exercises, their performance on spatial tasks improves.

Social Behavior

Aggression

Gender differences in the display of aggressive behavior first appear between ages 2 and 3, and persist across the life span. Boys engage in more overt physical aggression, especially during adolescence, whereas girls are more indirect, displaying hostility and verbal aggression. Meta-analyses indicate differences are greatest in situations where social expectations for males and females either endorse or restrict physical behavior (Eagly and Steffen, 1986). Physical aggression is related to power; men justify aggression when their superior status is being challenged. For women, physical aggression is about inflicting harm, not defending their status, making them more reluctant to fight.

A Social Class Perspective on Development

A Poverty rates by age and race

Category	No. (millions)	%
Persons	36.5	13.7
Age (< 18 yr)	14.5	20.5
Race—white	24.6	11.2
Race—black	9.7	28.4

B Child and poverty rates, 1959–1995

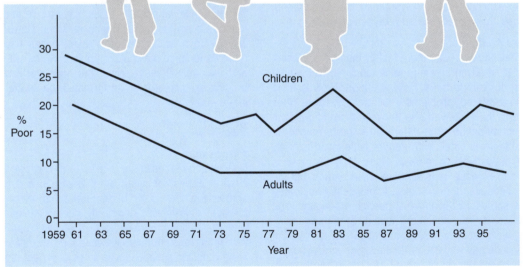

Any society exerts an enormous influence on the development of its members, and this influence is exerted in ways that are subtle but powerful. The latest census figures show that 36.5 million Americans live at or below the poverty level ($16,036 for a family of 4), and that African Americans, Hispanics, and women are overly represented in this group. The interaction of poverty, children, and education is a burning issue for our society, but first let's turn our attention to the extent of poverty itself.

The Culture of Poverty

Part A presents the total number of people living in poverty, by age and race. To summarize the statistics:

- Neither the number of poor nor the poverty rate for families showed significant changes between 1995 and 1996, which was true regardless of family type or race and ethnicity.
- In 1996, 14.4 million people had incomes of less than half of the poverty threshold, up from 13.9 million people in 1995.
- The number (10.6 million) and percentage (14.8) of uninsured children were statistically higher than the 1995 figures. An estimated 41.7 million (15.6%) Americans had no health insurance at all in 1996.

Although lack of an adequate income is what comes to mind when we think of poverty, it is important to remember that individuals and families living in poverty are extremely diverse. Many people visualize those in poverty as aging, alcoholic males; this is not the case. More young families and single women are living in poverty than ever before. The prevalence of poverty among women has reached a level, frequently referred to as the *feminization of poverty*. Health care providers often work with women on welfare, for example, and see the negative effects of poverty on pregnant women, both physically and psychologically.

Two reasons help explain the higher rate of children living in poverty compared to adults (see **Part B**). One reason is that poor families have more children per adult than the population as a whole does. For example, 55.7% of poor families with children have only 1 adult, but only 13.9% of nonpoor families with children have 1 adult. Another reason is that poor families with children have more children on average (2.24 per family) compared to nonpoor families with children (1.79) (Betson and Michael, 1997).

The Impact on Children

Poverty wreaks devastating effects on all aspects of development: physical, cognitive, and psychosocial. Americans have always been firm believers that schools are the means for students to turn their lives around. But today we must objectively ask, How good are the schools that these children attend? Jonathan Kozol, an outspoken critic of America's schools, wrote a biting commentary on classroom conditions in schools mostly attended by poor children. Students are crowded into small, squalid spaces, and in some cities overcrowding is so bad that schools function in abandoned factories. In 1 school, students eat their lunches in what was once the building's boiler room. Reading classes are taught in what used to be a bathroom; there are no microscopes for science classes; one counselor serves 3,600 students in the elementary grades. In the high school of the same district, there is a single physics section for 2,200 students; 2 classes are being taught simultaneously in 1 classroom.

Economic differences among school systems are also reflected in access to educational technology, certainly 1 of the gateways to future success. Commitment to a technological education, however, requires a substantial investment for acquiring machines and software. Some schools, owing to fiscal restraints, may find it necessary to cut supplies and expense budgets, resulting in fewer and less-sophisticated machines and software available to their students. The resulting "technology gap" (the gulf between schools that can afford basic or more elaborate equipment and supplies and those that cannot) may well widen the already existing gap between quality of schooling for those students in poorer versus wealthier areas.

Finally, here are some characteristics of schools that have functioned successfully under difficult economic conditions:

- They place an emphasis on academic achievement.
- They manifest a capacity to react swiftly to the social and emotional needs of their students.
- The school atmosphere is safe and orderly, but not restrictive.
- They display an open and encouraging attitude toward active parental participation in the running of the school.
- A true partnership exists between school administrators and all staff personnel.
- They maintain a close relationship with the community, which furthers the achievements of students.

Implications for Health Care Providers

Poverty hurts children in a range of ways difficult to identify because the poor are *not* all alike. For example, the African-American youth living in an urban ghetto experiences a quite different set of problems than a malnourished, chronically diseased white child in Appalachia. Although about 8% of American children are poor for more than 6 years, more than 30% of children experience poverty at some time in their life.

Impoverished and homeless children experience numerous health problems, usually due to a lack of medical care. When working with children on welfare or from homeless shelters, you should look especially for such problems as anemia, nutritional deficiencies, and any signs of lead poisoning. With adolescents, you should be alert for signs of chemical abuse, sexually transmitted diseases (STDs), and early symptoms of pregnancy.

PART I: QUESTIONS

Directions: For each of the following questions, choose the **one best** answer.

1. Development is best explained by a model that

(A) concentrates on one aspect of development.

(B) uses behavior as its focus.

(C) includes biological, psychological, and social influences.

(D) restricts itself to the observable.

2. Humans have a remarkable potential for change, but resiliency has

(A) limitations.

(B) defined markers.

(C) unlimited capacity.

(D) known characteristics.

3. A 10-year-old girl peeks in her older sister's diary, but later feels guilty. She tells herself, "I shouldn't have done that. It wasn't right." According to Freud, what moral component of the personality is responsible for her feelings about her behavior?

(A) Id

(B) Ego

(C) Superego

(D) Preconscious

4. What is Freud's "pleasure principle?"

(A) The notion that unconscious forces govern our behavior is the pleasure principle.

(B) Childhood pleasures have a strong influence on adult personality.

(C) Individuals act to gratify instinctual desires and to avoid pain.

(D) Personality is shaped by how individuals indulge their sexual urges.

5. Erikson's theory of psychosocial development is based on

(A) the notion that the personality develops early in childhood.

(B) the premise that humans interact with an ever-widening circle of people.

(C) the need to avoid developmental crises.

(D) the idea that early social experiences determine later ones.

6. Which of the following crises in the life cycle is the cornerstone of Erikson's theory?

(A) Trust vs mistrust

(B) Autonomy vs shame and doubt

(C) Initiative vs guilt

(D) Identity formation vs identity diffusion

7. Which of the following refers to Piaget's universalist constructivist theory?

(A) Humans passively assimilate their understanding of the world.

(B) Humans construct reality through interactions with the environment.

(C) Humans have inborn schemata to help them understand the world.

(D) Humans construct reality by being acted on by the environment.

8. What is Piaget's definition of "adaptation?"

(A) Intelligence

(B) Assimilation and accommodation

(C) Ability to effectively negotiate environmental demands

(D) All of the above

9. In his explanation of cognitive development, Vygotsky stressed

(A) assimilation.

(B) social interactions.

(C) reinforcement.

(D) schema.

10. Vygotsky believed language gradually becomes _____ and directs behavior.

(A) structured

(B) pragmatic

(C) internalized

(D) reinforced

11. In Bronfenbrenner's model of human ecology, the school, neighborhood, and peer group belong in which system?

(A) Microsystem

(B) Mesosystem

(C) Exosystem

(D) Macrosystem

12. The American cultural value placed on the primacy of the biological family is an example of a(n)

(A) microsystem.

(B) mesosystem.

(C) exosystem.

(D) macrosystem.

13. Maslow believed that our needs are best seen as a(n)

(A) ellipse.

(B) hierarchy.

(C) interlocking circle.

(D) polygon.

14. Using our abilities to the limits of our potential refers to

(A) assimilation.

(B) accommodation.

(C) conditioning.

(D) self-actualization.

15. The environment responds to human behavior and either reinforces it or eliminates it. This theory is known as

(A) operant conditioning.

(B) classical conditioning.

(C) social cognitive learning.

(D) connectionism.

16. The importance of modeling is emphasized in

(A) operant conditioning.

(B) classical conditioning.

(C) social cognitive learning.

(D) connectionism.

17. It is important to remember that different is not

(A) unique.

(B) deficient.

(C) appreciated.

(D) diffuse.

18. _____ is a belief that interactions among all aspects of development require analysis.

(A) Piagetian psychology

(B) Operant conditioning

(C) Social cognitive learning

(D) Developmental contextualism

19. Which of the following is an example of between-group differences in gender research on language development?

(A) Girls develop language more rapidly than boys.

(B) Girls do better on subtests of anagrams, synonyms, speech production, and word knowledge.

(C) Although dyslexia is more common in boys, some girls develop dyslexia.

(D) Gender accounts for 1% of the variability in language development.

20. Research on aggression supports which of the following statements?

(A) Boys are more hostile than girls.

(B) For men, physical aggression is about inflicting harm.

(C) For women, physical aggression is about defending their social status.

(D) Physical aggression is related to perceptions of social power.

21. Which of the following is not associated with homelessness?

(A) Hunger and poor nutrition

(B) Developmental delays

(C) Health problems

(D) Lowered intelligence

22. A major characteristic of successful schools in poor economic locations is

(A) an emphasis on academic achievement.

(B) classroom television.

(C) building conditions.

(D) proximity to the center of the city.

PART I: ANSWERS AND EXPLANATIONS

1. The answer is C.

The complexity of development demands an explanatory model that recognizes the interactions among the multiple levels that shape growth and development. Explanations that concentrate on only 1 topic are not adequate.

2. The answer is A.

No one can tolerate intense stress indefinitely. The secrets of resiliency still elude researchers.

3. The answer is C.

Emerging around ages 3–5 years, the superego represents an internalization of social standards for good and bad behavior. It is the individual's way of policing his or her own behavior. The 10-year-old girl has internalized social standards for privacy, and feels guilty knowing she has willfully violated those standards.

4. The answer is C.

As the most primitive component of personality, the id is the seat of instinctual drives, especially sex, food, and aggression. Operating on the pleasure principle, the id seeks immediate gratification and wants to avoid physical and psychic pain. The drives for sex and aggression are particularly conflicted because they are subject to ambiguous social norms. Freud developed the concept of defense mechanisms, which humans use to protect the ego from unpleasant feelings, especially anxiety and guilt.

5. The answer is B.

Erikson recognized that the social environment plays a significant role in shaping a child's sense of self. His theory of psychosocial development is based on the premise that humans interact with an ever-widening circle of people, beginning with mother and ending with mankind. The 8 stages are marked by normative developmental crises, the resolution of which form the personality.

6. The answer is D.

Erikson's concept of the identity crisis in adolescence is the cornerstone of his theory. He believed that most adolescents go through a serious struggle in achieving a self-identity. The developmental struggle is to integrate childhood identifications with new biological urges, assumption of social roles, and recognition of one's abilities and limitations. Failure to form an identity may result in identity diffusion, of feeling like a nobody, with no sense of direction or commitment to a set of values.

7. The answer is B.

The term *universal constructivist* implies that all humans construct their understanding of the world in predictable ways. Humans are not passive organisms, but take an active role in their own development by acting on the physical environment. Thus Piaget believed that mental life in infancy begins with motor activity. The infant who swings an arm toward and finally grasps a toy is learning about controlling the body, the nature of objects, and the relationship between body and objects.

8. The answer is D.

To Piaget, the definition of intelligence *is* adaptation, i.e., an ability to effectively negotiate environmental demands. Adaptation consists of the dual processes of assimilation and accommodation. When people assimilate, they incorporate an experience into existing schemata and structures. "Oh, I know this. It's just like that." When they cannot fit an experience into existing schemata or structures, people must accommodate, that is, modify their way of thinking to fit the experience. Accommodation can be a lot of mental work, hence, the famous line "assimilate if you can, accommodate if you must."

9. The answer is B.

Vygotsky's belief in the power of social interactions to shape development distinguished his work from other theorists such as Piaget.

10. The answer is C.

For Vygotsky, egocentric speech becomes internalized and helps to direct behavior. Speech is seen as playing a central role in cognitive development.

11. The answer is B.

The microsystem of the family is embedded in mesosystems, which include community groups in general, such as the school, neighborhood, peer group, and church or other social organizations.

12. The answer is D.

The macrosystem represents the dominant beliefs and ideologies in the culture at large. Beliefs about children in the society at large influence child-rearing practices and government policies. For example, the cultural value placed on the primacy of the biological family has resulted in children spending years in foster homes, even when reunification with biological parents may not be in the child's best interests.

13. The answer is B.

Maslow believed that a hierarchy best represents humans' needs since satisfaction of one need leads to the next. Each need can be partially satisfied before the drive to satisfy the next begins.

14. The answer is D.

The highest goal for humans is to be actually doing what they could be doing (self-actualization). Otherwise, a sense of restlessness, of wondering will persist.

15. The answer is A.

Skinner's interpretation of learning rests on the power of the environment to shape behavior. Careful control of the environment supposedly leads to positive, even ideal, development.

16. The answer is C.

Bandura's work on social cognitive learning has led to increased acceptance of the use of models to shape development. Properly presented, modeling can be a powerful tool in leading to desired behavior.

17. The answer is B.

We are all different to someone else. Consequently, individuals shouldn't be judged by their appearance, language, etc.

18. The answer is D.

Modern developmental psychologists are turning away from theories that focus on 1 aspect of development. Instead they have turned to explanations that recognize and analyze the complexities of human development.

19. The answer is A.

In research, differences are addressed in several ways. One way is to distinguish between-group from within-group differences, group differences from individual differences, and differences that are statistically significant but of no practical importance. For example, girls develop language more rapidly than boys (between-group difference), but there is a lot of variation among girls regarding their performance on tests of different types of language ability, such as anagrams and word knowledge (within-group differences). Even though dyslexia is more common in boys than girls, some girls do develop dyslexia (individual differences). Gender accounts for 1% of the variability in language development. This is statistically significant, but not necessarily important enough to justify developing special interventions for boys.

20. The answer is D.

Boys engage in more overt physical aggression, especially during adolescence, whereas girls are more indirect, displaying hostility and verbal aggression. Physical aggression is related to perceptions of social power, with men perceiving that aggression is justified when their superior status is being challenged. For example, fighting among males is more about standing up for one's self than about inflicting harm. For women, physical aggression is about inflicting harm, not defending their status, making them more reluctant to fight.

21. The answer is D.

Social class can often lead to misperceptions. A person's intelligence is not reflected by social status.

22. The answer is A.

Research has demonstrated that a focus on achievement is a feature of successful schools in deprived areas. Almost any other characteristic is secondary.

PART II
Prenatal Development

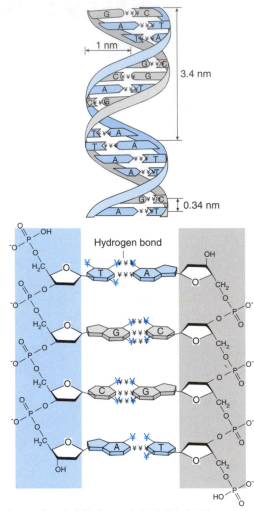

Source: Campbell, N., Reece, J., Mitchell, L. (1999).
Biology (5th ed.). Reading, MA: Addison Wesley Longman, Inc.

A basic understanding of genetics helps us to appreciate the complexity of human development, and the origins of some diseases. The information in genetic material is responsible for more than eye color. How a fetus develops in utero, how enzymes break down food, and how cancerous tumors grow are determined by, or at least influenced by, the instructions encoded in the DNA in the nucleus of the human body's cells.

DNA

The hereditary material carried in the nucleus of each somatic cell is called *deoxyribonucleic acid*, better known as *DNA*. In 1953, Watson and Crick, presented their model of the DNA molecule. It consisted of chemical compounds called *nucleotides*, linked together in two long chains that coiled to form a double helix.

Nucleotides consist of 3 subunits: a sugar molecule, a phosphate group, and 1 of 4 nucleotide bases. The bases of 1 chain in the double helix are linked to the bases of the other chain by hydrogen atoms, which hold the double helix together. The pairing of the bases is very specific. Adenine (A) and thymine (T) always link together, as do guanine (G) and cytosine (C), creating 4 possible complementary pairings: AT, TA, GC, and CG.

The double helix looks like a twisted ladder. The sequence of the nucleotide bases forms a long chain to make up each side of the ladder. The rungs of the ladder represent the pairings of the nucleotide bases between the chains (see **Part A**).

How can 4 possible pairs of nucleotide bases be enough? The key is the sequence in which they are arranged along and between the ladder, or double helix. The 3 billion base pairs in human DNA form an intricate code. The goal of the Human Genome Project (HGP) (see Chapter 16) is to identify the sequence of all of these pairs, to unlock the *genetic code*.

Function of DNA

DNA has 2 functions: transcription and translation. Transcription is the process by which DNA makes protein synthesis possible. The human body is composed of proteins. Some comprise the structural material for the human body (e.g., muscle, skin, blood cells), others (e.g., enzymes, hormones, insulin) regulate chemical reactions. If the body cannot synthesize proteins, it cannot live.

The contribution of DNA to protein synthesis works like this: Because DNA cannot leave the cell nucleus, it splits the double helix down the center, forming a single chain of nucleotides called *ribonucleic acid* or *messenger RNA* (*mRNA*). The mRNA transfers across the nuclear membrane into the cytoplasm. Because it acts as a template for DNA, mRNA transcribes information about the sequence of nucleic acids in DNA into the cell's *ribosomes*, which are the sites of protein synthesis. Any mistake in forming, transferring, or reading the mRNA template can cause protein synthesis to go awry, with potentially deadly consequences.

The sequence in which the nucleotide bases is arranged is crucial. A *code word*, also called a *codon*, refers to a specific arrangement of 3 bases, for example, ACG. There are 64 possible code words, which in different combinations are the genetic code for amino acids, the building blocks of proteins. There are 20 amino acids found in proteins. *Translation* is the process by which DNA replicates itself, passing a copy onto offspring, ensuring that human descendants have protein synthesizing information in their cells.

Genes

Each cell in the body contains about 6 feet of tightly coiled DNA. Just as multiple combinations of nucleic acids form code words, multiple combinations of code words along the DNA strand form genes. *Genes* are the functional units of DNA. Where and how in the longer strand of DNA they start and stop, and whether or not they overlap, depend on the careful placement of specific code words. Genes, sometimes alone, sometimes in combination, contain the coded information that determines particular traits in an individual person.

Chromosomes

Genes are arranged in linear order on *chromosomes*, which are long strands of DNA. Normal *somatic cells* (i.e., the cells that make up the major organs and body systems) contain 46 chromosomes arranged in 23 pairs of *homologous chromosomes*. One of each pair is inherited from each parent. Of the 23 pairs, 22 are autosomes, and 1 pair is the sex chromosomes.

Autosomes control most body traits, whereas the *sex chromosomes* determine gender as well as other traits. Females contain 2 X chromosomes: XX. Males contain 1 X and 1 Y chromosomes: XY.

Understanding Genetic Traits

Because of the homologous pairing of chromosomes, each person has 2 genes for each trait (e.g., eye color). However, they may or may not code for the same color. When genes have a variety of coded possibilities, they are called *alleles*. When you inherit 2 identical alleles, you are considered to be homozygous for that trait. When you inherit 2 different ones, you are heterozygous for the trait.

Which allele, or gene, determines eye color? *Dominant genes* prevail even when the paired allele has the code for a different variation on the trait. *Recessive genes* prevail only when both alleles are identical. For example, if you inherited 1 brown allele and 1 blue allele, you have brown eyes. Brown is the dominant gene. To have blue eyes, you must have inherited 2 blue alleles. Blue is the recessive gene. Two brown-eyed parents can have a blue-eyed child if both parents are heterozygous; that is, both have 1 brown allele and 1 blue allele. The child inherits the blue gene from each even though it was not expressed in either parent.

Genotype, Phenotype, and Disease

Each person's genetic code is called a *genotype*. How genotype is expressed is called *phenotype*. Two brown-eyed people have the same phenotype, but may have different genotypes, i.e., one may be heterozygous (brown/blue) and the other homozygous (brown/brown).

Phenotype is influenced by factors other than genes. For example, if you are genetically coded to be 6 feet tall but are malnourished in childhood, you may not reach your genetic potential. Similarly, certain diseases (e.g., hypertension) are polygenic in origin. When or if this genotype is expressed may depend on lifestyle habits, such as smoking, lack of exercise, and a diet rich in fats. Researchers suspect that a genotypic tendency for some cancers (e.g., Hodgkin's disease) may be triggered by viral infections.

12 Fertilization In Utero

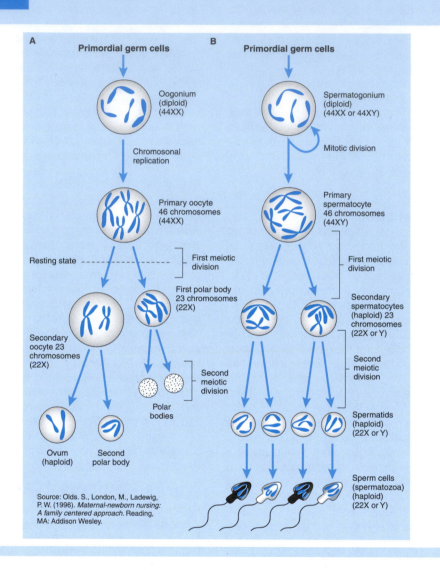

A   Primordial germ cells

Oogonium (diploid) (44XX)

Chromosonal replication

Primary oocyte 46 chromosomes (44XX)

Resting state — — — — — — — — — — — First meiotic division

First polar body 23 chromosomes (22X)

Secondary oocyte 23 chromosomes (22X)

Second meiotic division

Polar bodies

Ovum (haploid)   Second polar body

Source: Olds. S., London, M., Ladewig, P. W. (1996). *Maternal-newborn nursing: A family centered approach.* Reading, MA: Addison Wesley.

B   Primordial germ cells

Spermatogonium (diploid) (44XX or 44XY)

Mitotic division

Primary spermatocyte 46 chromosomes (44XY)

First meiotic division

Secondary spermatocytes (haploid) 23 chromosomes (22X or Y)

Second meiotic division

Spermatids (haploid) (22X or Y)

Sperm cells (spermatozoa) (haploid) (22X or Y)

Cell Development

Conception is the union of a sperm and an ovum, and marks the beginning of pregnancy. *Fertilization* is when 2 germ cells fuse to become 1 new cell, called the *zygote*. Germ cells are also called *gametes*. In females, they are *egg cells*, or *ova*. In males, they are *sperm cells*. Gametes develop through the process of cell division called meiosis.

Mitosis and Meiosis

Cells are produced by either mitosis or meiosis. Human somatic (body) cells are *diploid cells*; that is, they have 46 chromosomes arranged in 23 pairs. One pair carries the sex chromosomes, and is either XX or XY.

Mitosis is the process by which 1 diploid somatic cell divides to produce 2 diploid somatic cells identical to the original. The DNA in the chromosomes of the original cell replicates itself. After division, each new cell has 46 chromosomes.

Meiosis is the process of cell division by which 1 diploid somatic cell produces 4 haploid gamete cells. Haploid cells have half the number of chromosomes of the original diploid somatic cell, that is, 23 single chromosomes instead of 46 (see **Part A**).

There are 2 successive cell divisions in meiosis. First, the 46 chromosomes in the diploid somatic cell replicate. Then, rather than separate into 2 identical cells like in mitosis, the chromosomes intertwine and exchange genetic material. This exchange is responsible for genetic variability, such as eye color or height. When the cell divides, it forms 2 cells, each containing 23 chromosomes that are doubled in structure, but in combinations that are different from the original cell.

At the second division, the 23 double chromosomes split in half. The 2 halves, called chromatids, move apart, forming 2 more cells of 23 single chromosomes each. In other words, 4 different haploid cells arise from the original diploid cell.

Ovum

While the female fetus is still in utero, her ovarian somatic cells undergo meiosis to produce the gamete egg cells, or ova. Meiosis stops before the first division is complete. The cell, called the oocyte, contains 46 chromosomes, which have a doubled structure. The oocyte rests until puberty. All of a female's ova are in place by the sixth month of fetal life. A female infant is born with about 1 million egg cells, although half will no longer be viable by the time she reaches puberty.

At puberty, the oocyte divides into 2 cells, with 23 chromosomes, each with a doubled structure. One of the cells, the secondary oocyte, is larger and contains more cytoplasm than the smaller cell, the first polar body. The second meiotic division begins at ovulation. The first polar body divides into 2 smaller ones, which disintegrate. The secondary oocyte divides into a second polar body and immature ovum, each with 23 single chromosomes. This second division is not completed until fertilization, when the immature ovum forms a nucleus in response to penetration by sperm.

Sperm

Male gametes do not develop until puberty when cells in the testes undergo meiosis. After the second division, there are 4 haploid cells, called spermatids. Each has 23 chromosomes, 1 of which is either an X or a Y chromosome. A spermatid loses cytoplasm, its nucleus becomes compacted forming the head of the sperm, and a centriole develops into the tail. Sperm can remain viable in the testes for up to 42 hours.

Before Fertilization Occurs

Fertilization usually takes place in the outer third of the fallopian tubes. After the ovum is released, it is carried into the fallopian tubes by virtue of peristaltic movement caused by high estrogen levels. The ovum is surrounded by 2 membranes. The inner is the zona pellucida, which later nourishes the newly fertilized egg. The outer is the corona.

The mature ovum is fertile for 24 hours. Sperm can survive in the female reproductive tract for 72 hours. Of the 200–400 million sperm released during ejaculation, only 200 will reach the fallopian tubes in about 4 hours. Only 1 sperm may fertilize an ovum.

A sperm's success depends on several things. The head of the sperm is covered by a cap called the acrosome. First, the coating over the acrosomal cap is removed by enzymes in the female uterus.

Second, enzymes covering the acrosome are deposited on the outer membrane of the ovum. The enzymes break down the corona, allowing 1 sperm to penetrate into the ovum's zona pellucida.

The ovum may be selective about which sperm it allows in, and may engulf the sperm, drawing it in.

The Moment of Fertilization

As the sperm enters the ovum, cellular changes in the zona pellucida block other sperm from entering. Then meiotic division in the ovum is completed, as the mature ovum develops a nucleus, and the second polar body is ejected.

Immediately, the newly developed nuclei of the ovum and the nuclei of the sperm move toward each other. Their individual nuclei each contain 23 single chromosomes, the haploid number. The nuclei membranes disappear, allowing the chromosomes to pair up, resulting in 46 chromosomes, arranged in 23 pairs. This transformation results in the zygote, a diploid somatic cell that contains all of the genetic material for an individual who will be different from either parent . . . and from everyone else.

Gender is determined at the moment of fertilization. A mature ovum can only carry the X chromosome. However, a sperm cell may carry either the X or the Y chromosome on its 23rd chromosome. Thus, the sex chromosome carried by the sperm determines the gender of the human organism. A pairing of XX results in a female child; XY results in a boy.

Implications for Health Care Providers

For every 100 ova exposed to sperm, 84 are fertilized, 69 are implanted, 42 survive 1 week, 37 survive to 7 weeks prenatally, and 31 survive to birth. That is, there is a 70% rate of spontaneous abortion (i.e., miscarriage) prenatally.

More males are conceived than females, in a ratio of 160 to 105. But more male embryos die in utero, so that at birth the male-female ratio is 105 to 100. Boys are more vulnerable than girls, and by age 18, the genders are equally represented in the population.

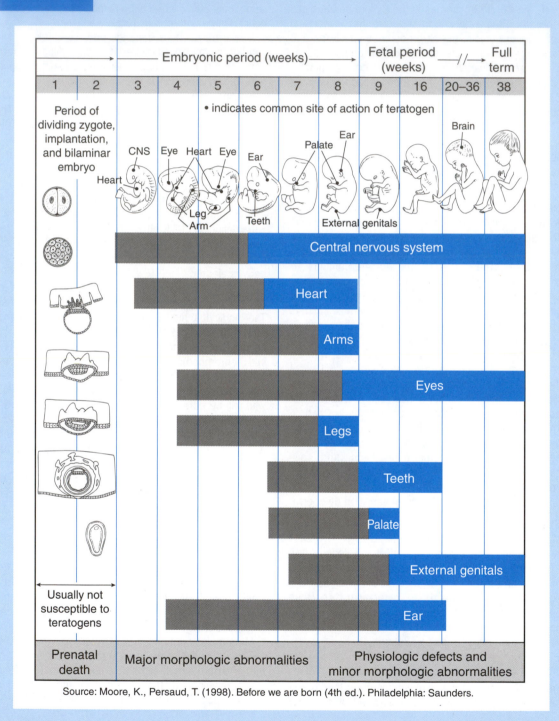

Source: Moore, K., Persaud, T. (1998). Before we are born (4th ed.). Philadelphia: Saunders.

Understanding prenatal development is important for 2 reasons. First, the developing organism is open to environmental influences over a period of 40 weeks. The timing and nature of these influences can permanently alter the development of the fetus. Second, how development occurs prior to birth gives us information about development after birth.

Embryonic Development: 0–8 Weeks

Embryo is the name given to the fertilized ovum during the first 8 weeks of prenatal development. The first 2 weeks are also called the germinal period. From 3 to 8 weeks is the critical period of organogenesis, during which all of the major organs develop (see **Part A**).

Germinal Period: 0–2 Weeks

0–40 hours: The fertilized ovum is called the zygote, and consists of 2–4 cells. It rests in the fallopian tube.

40–72 hours: Having grown to 12–16 cells, the morula floats into the uterus, and grows to 64 cells.

4–8 days: The blastocyst continues to grow to over 100 cells. The inner cell mass becomes the human organism itself. The trophoblast forms between the inner mass and the environment, and will later develop into the placenta. By day 6 or 7, the blastocyst implants on the uterine wall, or endometrium, a process called nidation.

8–13 days: Cells separate and arrange themselves into 3 embryonic germ layers, which give rise to all of the major organs. (1) The ectoderm—outer layer—gives rise to the nervous system (including the brain and spine), skin, nails, hair, and salivary, pituitary, and mammary glands. (2) The endoderm—innermost layer—gives rise to the thyroid, bladder, lungs, and digestive system. (3) The mesoderm—which emerges between the ectoderm and endoderm—gives rise to the heart, circulatory and lymph systems, connective tissue, muscle, and bones. By the end of the second week, the placenta, umbilical cord, and amniotic sac have taken shape.

Period of the Embryo: 3–8 Weeks

Third week: An indentation of cells, called the neural plate, forms in the ectoderm, giving rise to the brain (hindbrain, midbrain, forebrain) and neural tube (spinal cord). The chambers of the heart and blood vessels arise from a similar process in the mesoderm.

Fourth week: The heart begins to beat. Limb buds are visible. Eyes, ears, nerves, and the skeletomuscular and digestive systems begin to form. Vertebrae are present; major veins and arteries are completed. The neural tube closes. The embryo is about 0.5 cm long and weighs 0.4 g.

Fifth week: Bronchial buds form, and will become the lungs. Hand plates form.

Sixth week: Sex differentiation occurs. The head becomes prominent, the lower jaw fuses, and the parts of the upper jaw are present. The external ear is visible.

Seventh week: The face, eyelids, and neck form. The stomach is in position. Muscles are forming throughout the body, and neurons are developing at the rate of thousands per minute.

Eighth week: The head is elevated so that the neck is distinct. The inner and middle ear develop. The embryo moves and responds to some stimulation. Ninety-five percent of organogenesis is complete. The human organism is about 2–3 cm long and weighs 2 g. The mother is probably now aware that she is pregnant.

Fetal Development: 10–40 Weeks

Fetus is the name given to the prenatal human organism from 2 months to birth.

10–12 weeks: The intestines are in position, the spinal cord is apparent, eyes take final form, and blood forms in bone marrow. Sex organs appear. Urine forms. The fetus is 6–8 cm long and weighs 19 g.

16 weeks: The fetus looks human. Bones and joints are distinct; the 2 halves of the brain are visible. The hard and soft palate of the mouth are differentiated. Lanugo (fine hair) and vernix caseosa (oil) begin to appear on skin. The fetus is 12 cm long and weighs 100 g.

20 weeks: Dental enamel forms. All of the nerve cells a person will have for life are present. Sheathing of nerve fibers begins, but will not be complete until many years later. The fetus is active, kicking, sucking, and sleeping. The heartbeat is audible. The intestines work. The fetus is 16–18 cm long and weighs 300 g.

24 weeks: Fat begins to accumulate under the skin. Fetal activity slows as higher regions of the brain form, quieting fetal reflexes in response to random stimuli. The eyes are complete. The fetus is 23 cm long and weighs 600 g.

28 weeks: Fetal activity increases again as brain develops. Growth slows, and fat forms beneath the skin. Fingernails appear. The eyes open, close, and respond to light. Surfactant begins to form in the lungs, allowing them to expand without collapsing. The fetus is viable, capable of breathing. The fetus is 27 cm long and weighs 1,100 g.

32 weeks: Fetus responds to external sounds. Testes descend into the scrotum. Fetus looks smooth and chubby, and should be in a head-down position for delivery. The brain is 25% of its adult weight. The fetus is 31 cm long and weighs 1,800–2,100 g.

36 weeks: The fetus adds 50% of its birth weight in the last month. Growth slows and the brain becomes more convoluted, although the cerebral cortex does not yet influence volitional behavior. Lanugo hair disappears.

By 40 weeks: The fetus has smooth skin, moderate to profuse hair on its head, and lanugo hair on the shoulders only. Myelination of the brain begins. The fetus is 40 cm and weighs 3,200 g.

14 Infertility

A

Myth	Fact
Infertility is a woman's problem.	Infertility is a female problem in 35% of the cases, a male problem in 35% of the cases, a shared problem in 20% of the cases, and unexplained in 10% of the cases.
Fertilization is not really a problem.	More that 5 million people of childbearing age in the United States experience infertility.
Fertilization is more of a mental than a physical problem.	Infertility is a disease or disorder of the reproductive system. Psychological factors may be responsible, but only in a small number of cases.
Is the couple doing something wrong?	Infertility is a medical condition, not a sexual disorder.

B

Male	Female
Environmental	Ovulation problems
Sperm count	Tubal blockage
Sperm interactions	Endometriosis
Infections	IUDs
Varicocele	Voluntary
Structural	Other
Voluntary	

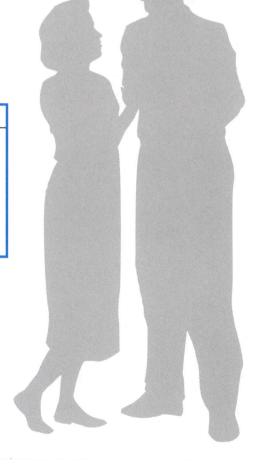

For nonprofessionals, *infertility* probably means an inability to have children. Unfortunately, it is not that simple. A couple may easily conceive their first child, but have difficulty conceiving again. A couple who had conceived with previous partners may not be able to conceive together. Estimates are that about 1 in 5 or 6 American couples meet the criteria for infertility: an inability to achieve pregnancy after 2 years.

Table A presents the myths and facts about infertility.

Causes of Infertility

The causes of infertility can be traced to either the man or the woman (see **Table B**).

Possible Causes of Male Infertility

Fertility specialists have concluded that male infertility has increased in the last 50 years (especially in Western countries) and have turned their suspicions to a wide range of agents.

- **Environment.** Environmental pollutants such as polychlorinated biphenyls (PCBs) may be partly responsible for reduced male fertility. Other environmental agents such as nicotine, alcohol, marijuana, and stress are also associated with a lowered sperm count and defective sperm.
- **Sperm count.** Lower sperm count alone (<20 million sperm/mL) is *not* a cause of infertility. Many men with a low sperm count father children, although it may take a longer time. On rare occasions, a man's semen may lack sperm due to a congenital problem with the testes, or even because of a blow to the testes. Infections can also cause this condition. Other male problems include premature ejaculation, retrograde ejaculation, impotence, and an inability to sustain an erection.
- **Varicocele.** Varicocele is a condition in which valves in the veins that carry blood away from the testicles do not function properly. As a result, blood pools around the testicles and generates extra heat near the sperm production centers, thus reducing the number of sperm.
- **Structural problems.** About 10% of male infertility is due to difficulties in the sperm transport system. The passage of sperm is blocked, usually because of previous infections. Surgery is typically required to remove the blockage.
- **Voluntary infertility.** Estimates are that 500,000 vasectomies are performed each year in the United States. The resulting sterility is generally permanent due to the difficulty of reversing the procedure.
- **Sperm interactions.** Once a man's sperm has been judged healthy, attention focuses on what happens to the sperm once they enter the vagina. Do the sperm penetrate the cervical mucus? Are there any antibodies present in the cervical mucus that attack the sperm? Does the head of the sperm possess the necessary enzymes that permit the sperm to penetrate the outer membrane of the egg?

Possible Causes of Female Infertility

When a woman is unable to conceive, the initial search for causes usually turns to the timing and functioning of her menstrual cycle.

- **Ovulation problems.** If luteinizing hormone (LH) and follicle-stimulating hormone (FSH) are not secreted in proper proportions, mature eggs may not form. Occasionally, scarring due to previous surgery on ovarian cysts or the effects of radiation treatment damage the ovary, resulting in diminished egg production.
- **Tubal blockage.** The fallopian tubes, which ensnare eggs when they are released from the ovary, may be blocked. If blockage occurs, sperm cannot travel through the tube to meet and fertilize the egg. One of the most common causes of tubal blockage is an STD, especially infection with chlamydia, usually a silent infection that may lurk in a woman's pelvic organs. STDs can lead to *pelvic inflammatory disease* (PID), which can cause infertility. About 30% of infertility problems in women are due to tubal blockage.
- **Endometriosis.** About 15% of all women have endometriosis, a condition in which the growth of endometrial tissue occurs outside of the uterus.
- **Intrauterine devices (IUDs).** Although discredited because of the hazards they introduce, especially the risk of infection, they still are responsible for some problems seen today.
- **Voluntary infertility.** For women, sterilization takes the form of blocking or cutting the fallopian tubes to prevent passage of the egg to the uterus.
- **Other causes.** If the cervical mucus is too thick or contains antibodies that attack the sperm, then fertilization is impossible. The uterus, its shape, condition, and susceptibility to fibroids (benign tumors) can occasionally cause fertility problems (see **Table**).

Implications for Health Care Providers

Determining infertility requires time, effort, and careful examination by a fertility specialist. You can help couples clarify their status by posing several questions:

- How long have they attempted to conceive and how frequent were their attempts?
- Have either of them conceived any children?
- Do they smoke or drink? Have they ever taken drugs? What medications have they been on? What illnesses and operations have they had?

15 Assisted Reproductive Techniques

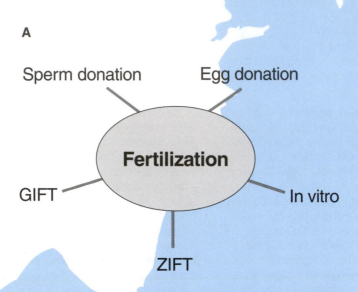

A

Sperm donation

Egg donation

Fertilization

GIFT

In vitro

ZIFT

B

Name	Meaning
Gamete intrafallopian transfer (GIFT)	Sperm and egg are placed in the fallopian tube, a more natural environment for fertilization.
Zygote intrafallopian transfer (ZIFT)	The fertilized egg is transferred to the fallopian tube.
Cryopreservation	Embryos are frozen for future use.
Surrogacy	One woman carries another woman's embryo to term.

Although there is about a 90% chance of diagnosing the causes of infertility, the problem can't always be corrected. Before adopting any assisted reproductive technology (ART), couples need thoughtful analysis, extensive research, and considerable caution. (**Part A** illustrates several assisted reproductive techniques.)

Common ART Procedures

Sperm Donation

When a couple determines that the problem is related to sperm, they have several choices.

- **Artificial insemination by partner (AIP).** AIP is when a woman is inseminated with her partner's sperm. Sperm is introduced into the cervical canal or uterus, thus avoiding any potential problems with vaginal fluids.
- **Donor insemination.** Artificial insemination by donor sperm, or donor insemination, is more frequent than AIP when the partner's sperm count is low, when the male partner is sterile, or when there is a background of genetic disorders, or Rh incompatibility.
- **Sperm banks.** The appeal of this technique lies in the screening processes used, which are intended to reduce the risk of STDs. In 1985, mandatory screening of donors for the human immunodeficiency virus (HIV) and freezing and quarantining of semen became required, and since then, to the best of our knowledge, no women have been infected with HIV through donor insemination (Marrs et al., 1997).

The donor's traits are carefully recorded, since most couples want to match the male partner's characteristics as closely as possible. Donors typically receive a fee of about $100 and are not told about the use of their sperm. They must also waive all parental rights to any children conceived with their sperm.

In Vitro Fertilization

In vitro fertilization (IVF) is the more commonly known fertilization technique. The steps are as follows.

1. The woman is usually treated with hormones to stimulate maturation of eggs in the ovary, and she is observed closely to determine the timing of ovulation (i.e., the time at which the egg leaves the surface of the ovary).
2. The physician makes an incision in the abdomen and inserts a laparoscope (a thin tubular lens through which the physician can see the ovary) to remove mature eggs.
3. The egg is placed in a solution containing blood serum and nutrients.
4. Capacitation, a process in which a layer surrounding the sperm is removed so that it may penetrate the egg, takes place.
5. Sperm are added to the solution and fertilization occurs.
6. The fertilized egg is transferred to a fresh supporting solution.
7. Fertilized eggs (usually 3) are inserted into the uterus.
8. The fertilized egg is implanted in the uterine lining.

During the IVF process, the woman is treated with hormones to prepare her body to receive the fertilized egg. About 27,000 IVF procedures are done every year in the United States with an estimated success rate at about 20% (Marrs et al., 1997).

Egg Donation

If a woman is unable to produce an egg, a donor's egg may be used for IVF. Donor eggs are not widely available, however, and usually come from relatives or IVF patients who donate their extra eggs. This in itself may be a problem because many women using IVF techniques are older, raising the possibility of chromosomal disorders in their egg cells. Also, a woman having difficulty with egg production may not have a particularly receptive uterine lining.

Timing is again critical here because uterine development must precisely match the ovarian cycle and ovulation for implantation to occur. The difficulty is increased when 2 women are involved. To solve the timing problem, the donor woman receives drug treatment to slow her ovulation time in an attempt to match the development of the uterine lining of the woman receiving the donor egg. When the match seems ideal, ovulation is triggered in the donor and her eggs are harvested, fertilized with the male partner's sperm, and inserted into the receiving woman's uterus.

Other ARTs

Many new forms of ART are now available (see **Part B**). Consequently, today a child may have as many as five parents: a sperm donor (father or other male), an egg donor (mother or other female), a surrogate mother, the couple who raise the child. These new techniques raise critical legal and ethical issues.

Implications for Health Care Providers

Couples who turn to ART usually have been diagnosed with one or more of the fertility problems discussed in Chapter 14 and typically are experiencing emotional turmoil. When working with these individuals, encourage them to learn as much as possible about their infertility problem, which helps them to feel they have input into the process. Be alert for any signs of blame or guilt and urge both partners to discuss matters with you, thus helping to maintain a positive relationship. Above all, impress on both partners the importance of not letting the infertility crisis take over their lives. Keep in mind that the time may come when you feel the necessity of recommending professional counseling (Marrs et al., 1997).

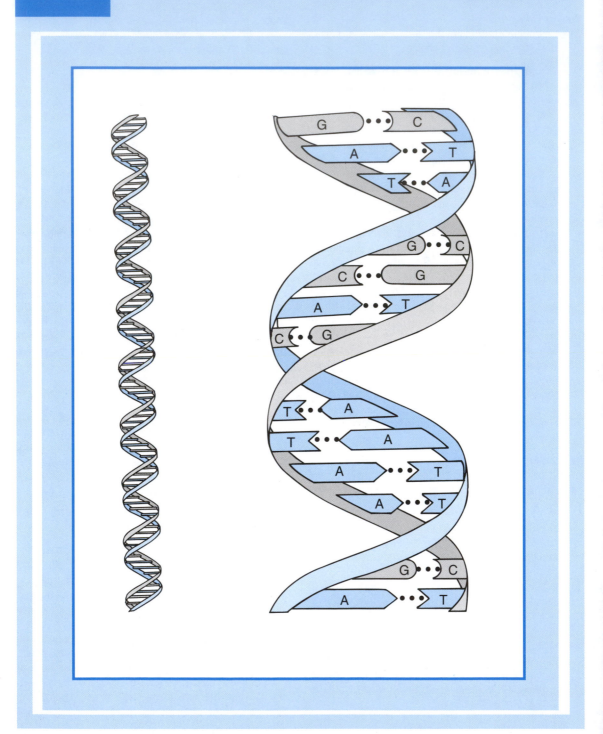

On June 26, 2000, Dr. Francis Collins (Director of the National Human Genome Research Institute) and Dr. J. Craig Venter (President of Celera Genomics) announced at a White House ceremony that they had completed a "rough draft of the human genome." The Human Genome Project has been nothing less than an attempt to identify and map the 50,000 to 100,000 genes that constitute our genetic makeup (Cohen, 1997; Hart, 2000). Because it requires over 3 billion chemical letters (A, T, C, G) to identify the DNA instructions by which an individual develops from an embryo to an adult, you can understand the immensity of the project.

How the Human Genome Project Began

Two gatherings of America's top biologists in the 1980s are credited as the forerunners of the project. In 1985, a group of scientists met at the University of California, Santa Cruz to discuss the possibility of mapping the human genome. (A *genome* is all the genetic material in a human chromosome.) Most of the participants at this meeting were sure it could be done, but were skeptical that it should be done because of the enormous expense. Because of the widespread benefits that would come from the project, however, almost all of the scientists present agreed that it deserved continued consideration. In March of the following year, a meeting of international scientists took place in Santa Fe, New Mexico. This meeting is considered to be the actual beginning of the HGP. The National Institutes of Health (NIH), with the assistance of the Department of Energy (DOE), assumed leadership of the project.

The Goals

Francis Collins, the director of the NIH HGP, has identified its continuing objectives as follows:

- Continued mapping of the human genome, that is, mapping the 100,000 genes present in each chromosome.
- Identification of all the genes in the genome.
- Advance DNA sequencing. (Sequencing is the process of determining the order of the nucleotides—A, T, C, and G—along a DNA strand.)
- Development of new and improved technologies.
- Continued investigation of the ethical, social, and legal aspects of the project.

These goals are elusive, which is understandable when you realize that genes make up only 3% of DNA. (Scientists call the remaining 97% "evolutionary junk.")

The Accomplishments to Date

To address the accomplishments to date, we turn to the Genome Database, a public repository for human genome mapping information. Among the more significant achievements of the HGP are the following:

- As of January 20, 1998, about 6,000 genes have been identified.

- The physical mapping of the genes continues unabated and now shows about 8,000 landmarks. More detailed maps have been produced for individual chromosomes. These maps help researchers unlock the secrets of many diseases and will play an integral role in the battle against such complex disorders as cancer, heart disease, and psychiatric problems. For example, investigators recently discovered that 5 different chromosomes play a role in insulin-dependent diabetes.
- Roughly 2.5% of the human genome has been sequenced. Significant advances have been made in improving the sequencing technology. Knowing the order of the nucleotides on the DNA helps researchers to discover where genes are located and to determine what instructions are carried in the DNA. These discoveries are central to understanding the function of genes and how they cause disease.

These achievements have had a dramatic impact. The genes responsible for cystic fibrosis and Huntington's disease have been identified, as has a gene abnormality that causes some cases of Parkinson's disease. Scientists from the NIH found that 3 specific alterations in the breast cancer genes BRCA1 and BRCA2 are associated with an increased risk of breast, ovarian, and prostate cancer. Although the risk of cancer is higher for these individuals than for those without the alterations, the risk is actually lower than earlier estimates.

In spite of these successes, the difficulty of the task that remains cannot be discounted. Although there are hundreds of diseases caused by a single gene, for thousands of others the contribution is much more obscure. For example, some diseases (e.g., possibly diabetes) need an environmental trigger, whereas for other diseases more than one gene may have to be faulty.

Studies of genetic susceptibility will undoubtedly follow the same pattern. The genes that make people susceptible to certain diseases do not, by themselves, cause disease. Rather, the combination of a particular environmental factor with a particular gene is needed. Once the mechanisms that cause a susceptibility gene to spring into action are more fully understood, such preventative measures as screening techniques and drug therapy will save many lives.

Implications for Health Care Providers

Several ethical, legal, and social issues (ELSI) demand your attention. Unfortunately, this explosion of knowledge is also leading to uncertain, even dangerous, consequences. For example, if a family member is susceptible to a particular disease, do insurance companies have the legal right to deny this person, and perhaps the entire family, health insurance? How private or public is a person's medical history? Grappling with this and similar issues has led to the creation of a program for studying the ethical, legal, and social implications of the HGP—the *ELSI* program.

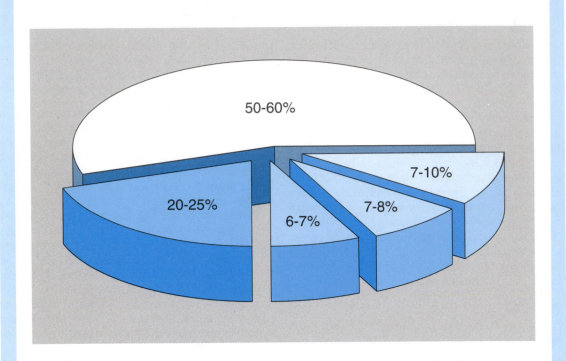

Unknown etiology

Multifactorial inheritance

Chromosomal abnormalities

Mutant genes

Environmental agents

Genes reproduce themselves, but as cells divide, the genes do not remain identical. Specialization occurs and different kinds of cells are formed at different locations. In the process, mistakes happen, leading to defects and disorders that affect normal function. In 1996 the primary cause of infant deaths was congenital abnormalities, accounting for 6,463 infant deaths.

Genetic Abnormalities

This section discusses the incidence and characteristics of several specific genetic disorders.

Tay-Sachs Disease

Jews of Eastern European origin are struck hardest by Tay-Sachs disease, which causes death by the age of 4 or 5 years. At birth, the afflicted children appear normal, but development slows by the age of 6 months, and mental and motor deterioration begin. About 1 in every 25–30 Jews of Eastern European origin carries the defective gene, which is recessive; thus danger arises when 2 carriers marry. The disease results from a gene failing to produce an enzyme that breaks down fatty materials in the brain and nervous system. The result is that fat accumulates and destroys nerve cells, causing loss of coordination, blindness, and finally death.

Sickle-cell Anemia

Sickle-cell anemia mainly affects people of African descent, appeared thousands of years ago in equatorial Africa, and increased resistance to malaria. Estimates are that 10% of the African-American population in the United States carry the sickle-cell trait. Thus, 2 carriers of the defective gene who marry have a 1 in 4 chance of producing a child with sickle-cell anemia. In patients with sickle-cell anemia, the red blood cells are distorted and pointed. Because of the cells' shape, they encounter difficulty in passing through the blood vessels. They tend to pile up and clump, producing oxygen starvation accompanied by considerable pain. The body then acts to eliminate these cells, and anemia results.

Cystic Fibrosis (CF)

In the population of the United States, CF is the most severe genetic disease of childhood, affecting about 1 in 1,200 children. About 1 in 30 individuals is a carrier. The disease causes a malfunction of the exocrine glands, the glands that secrete tears, sweat, mucus, and saliva. Breathing and digestion are difficult because of the thickness of the mucus. The secreted sweat is extremely salty, often producing heat exhaustion. CF has killed more children than any other genetic disease but the CF gene now has been identified, and new research offers hope concerning the detection of carriers.

Phenylketonuria (PKU)

PKU results from the body's failure to break down the amino acid phenylalanine, which then accumulates, affects the nervous system, and causes mental retardation. Most states now require infants to be tested at birth. If phenylalanine is present in the blood, the infants are placed on a special diet that has been remarkably successful.

However, success has produced other problems. Women treated successfully as infants may give birth to children with mental retardation because of a toxic uterine environment. Thus at the first signs of pregnancy, these women must return to a special diet. The person cured of phenylketonuria still carries the faulty genes.

Spina Bifida

Spina bifida (failure of the spinal column to close completely) is an example of a genetic defect caused by the interaction of several genes with possible environmental factors. It affects about 1 in 1,000 births, depending on geographic location. If the embryo's neural tube does not close, spina bifida results, causing mental retardation and paralysis of the lower limbs. Studies have shown that if a woman takes extra folic acid while she is pregnant, the risk for spina bifida decreases (Blackman, 1997).

Sex-linked Disorders

Disorders also occur because of what is known as sex-linked inheritance. The X chromosome is substantially larger than the Y chromosome, and the female carries more genes on the 23rd chromosome than does the male. This difference helps to explain sex linkage. Think back now to the difference between dominant and recessive traits. If a dominant and a recessive gene appear together, the dominant trait is expressed. An individual must have 2 recessive genes for the recessive trait (e.g., blue eyes) to appear. But on the 23rd set of chromosomes, nothing on the Y chromosome offsets any negative effects of a gene on the X chromosome.

Perhaps the most widely known of these sex-linked disorders is hemophilia, a condition in which the blood does not clot properly. Several of the royal families of Europe were particularly prone to this condition. Another sex-linked trait attributed to the X chromosome is color blindness. The X chromosome contains the gene for color vision and if it is faulty, nothing on the Y chromosome counterbalances the defect.

18 Chromosomal Abnormalities

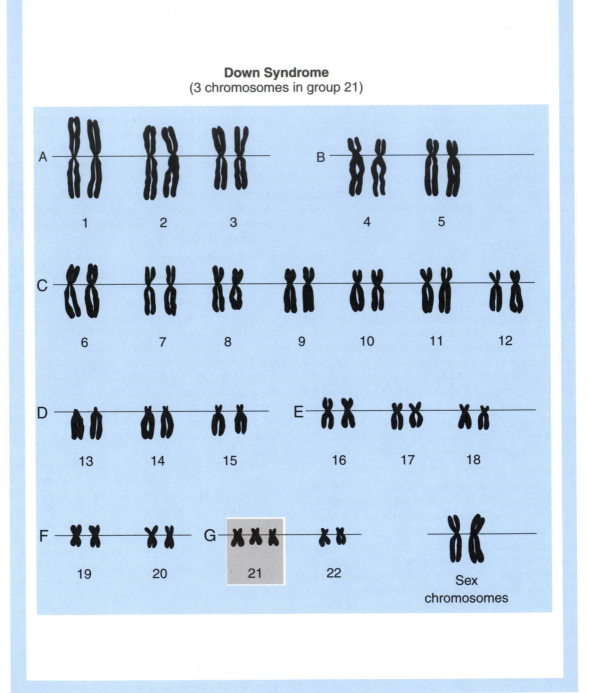

Down Syndrome
(3 chromosomes in group 21)

Chromosomal Abnormalities

Chromosomal abnormalities usually fall into one of two categories. One category, *abnormalities of number*, includes individuals born with too many or too few chromosomes. An example of an abnormality due to too many chromosomes is trisomy 21, in which an individual has an extra chromosome, producing a total of 47 chromosomes, the well-known *Down syndrome*. This defect was discovered in 1866 by a British doctor, Langdon Down, and produces distinctive facial features, small hands, small oral cavity, and possible functional difficulties such as mental retardation, heart defects, and an increased risk of leukemia.

The appearance of Down syndrome is closely related to the mother's age: Chances of giving birth to a child with Down syndrome are about 1 in 750 between the ages of 30 and 35; 1 in 300 between ages 35 and 39; and 1 in 80 between ages 40 and 45. After age 45 years the incidence jumps to 1 in 40 births. Before age 30 the ratio is only 1 in 1,500 births. Recent evidence suggests that in one-third of Down syndrome children, the extra chromosome may come from the father (Blackman, 1997).

Other disorders relate to the sex chromosomes. Estimates are that 1 in every 1,200 females and 1 in every 400 males have some disorder in the sex chromosomes. Occasionally a male will possess an XXY pattern rather than the normal XY. This disorder, called *Klinefelter's syndrome*, may cause small testicles, reduced body hair, possible infertility, and language impairment. Klinefelter's syndrome occurs in about 1 in 1,000 male births. Another pattern that may appear in males is XYY (about 1 in 1,000 male births), causing larger size and increased aggression.

Females occasionally possess an XO pattern (lack of a chromosome, resulting in 45 chromosomes) rather than XX. This is called *Turner's syndrome* (occurring in about 1 in 2,500 female births) and is characterized by short stature, poorly developed secondary sex features (such as breast size), and usually sterility.

The second category of chromosomal disorders, *abnormalities of structure*, refers to the loss or gain of parts of chromosomes because of breaking or rejoining. For example, certain spots on chromosomes are especially prone to breakage. The tip of the long arm of the X chromosome seems particularly fragile. A break here is called the fragile X syndrome. Estimates are that about 1 in 166 newborns has a chromosomal abnormality.

Implications for Health Care Providers

Here are several risk factors to keep in mind during your clinical work.

- **Advanced parental age.** Maternal age older than 35 and paternal age older than 50 are associated with an increased risk for chromosomal abnormalities.
- **History of miscarriages or stillbirths.** Couples who have experienced 3 or more miscarriages may carry a chromosomal problem that predisposes to miscarriage and chromosomal abnormalities in their children.
- **Previous children with birth defects, mental retardation, growth retardation, or neurological problems.** Any of these conditions may be an isolated event or an indicator of chromosomal or genetic disorders.
- **Family history of birth defects.** A carefully researched family history is important. Some couples needlessly worry about the possibility of a disorder arising or conversely, ignore potential problems because of inadequate information.
- **Exposure to medications, radiation, or toxic chemicals.** Exposure to any teratogenic agent caucauses concern about the chances of abnormalities occurring.
- **Ethnic background.** Certain groups are more susceptible to specific genetic disorders.

Influences on Prenatal Development

Prescription Medications during Pregnancy

The use of prescription medications during pregnancy is referred to as a managed risk. The decision to use a medication is made by weighing the benefits to the mother against the risks to the fetus, especially during the first trimester of gestation (see Table). The Food and Drug Administration has developed a classification system for all medications (categories A, B, C, D, and X) that can be found in any pharmacology reference book.

Medication (Use)	Effects on Fetus and Neonate
Benefit outweighs risk	
Aspirin (pain)	Malformations of the CNS, bones, and internal organs
Insulin (diabetes mellitus)	Malformation of the sacrum (lower spine)
Isoniazid (tuberculosis)	Increase of anomalies
Glucocorticoids, e.g., prednisone (antiinflammatory)	Cleft palate, cardiac defects
Penicillin (infections)	No known adverse effect
Benefit vs risk uncertain	
Lithium (bipolar disorder)	Cleft palate, anomalies of the eye, goiter
Cytotoxic drugs (cancer) trimethoprim-sulfamethoxazole	Increase of anomalies
Sulfonamides, e.g., Septra (antiinfective)	Cleft palate
Aminoglycosides, e.g., gentamicin (antiinfective)	8th cranial nerve damage (hearing)
Risk outweighs benefit	
Tetracycline (antibiotic)	Inhibited bone growth, discolored teeth in childhood
Methotrexate (cancer, arthritis)	Multiple anomalies; has been used as an abortive
Warfarin (i.e., Coumadin) (blood thinner)	Skeletal and facial anomalies, mental retardation
Iodide (hypothyroidism)	Congenital goiter, mental retardation

Whatever affects the mother can affect the fetus. Potentially harmful extrauterine influences are called teratogens (from *teras* for "monster," *genesis* for "origin") because of the sometimes devastating affects on the child.

The relationship between the timing of prenatal exposure to a teratogen and fetal development is critical. Exposure from the third to eighth week—when 95% of major organ systems form—can result in major abnormalities of vital structures, such as arms, legs, heart, and eyes. Later exposure may cause organs to malfunction. Long-term exposure (e.g., to alcohol) is most devastating of all. The effects are usually both irreversible and preventable.

Chemical Substances

Alcohol interferes with fetal cell division and growth throughout pregnancy. During the third trimester in particular, alcohol adversely alters development of the central nervous system (CNS) and brain. *Fetal alcohol syndrome* is found in about 40% of infants born to alcoholics. It is characterized by retarded growth before and after birth; unusual facial features, such as a small head, flat philtrum (no depression between the nose and upper lip), and small widely spaced eyes; and structural abnormalities of the palate, heart, kidneys, and bladder. The most striking deficit is impaired intellectual capacity, especially mental retardation, often accompanied by seizures. Withdrawal from alcohol causes tremors, increased muscle tone, and irritability.

Cocaine increases maternal and fetal heart rates and blood pressures, decreases blood flow to the fetus, and causes uterine contractions. Complications include fetal death, spontaneous abortion, premature birth, infants small for gestational age (SGA), and ventricular hemorrhage (i.e., bleeding into the brain). Infants also experience abnormalities of the genitourinary system and neurological irritability, such as disturbed wake-sleep cycles, increased muscle tone, difficulty being soothed, and learning disabilities.

Smoking decreases blood flow to the placenta, constricts blood vessels in the uterus, and interferes with maternal absorption of vitamins and calcium. Mothers who smoke, especially older mothers, have a higher incidence of premature birth and placenta previa (separation from the uterine wall). Their full-term infants are more likely to have a lower birth weight.

Medications pregnant women use are also chemial substances (**Part A**).

Infectious Diseases

The most common diseases that are potentially harmful to the fetus are referred to by the acronym STORCH: syphilis, toxomoplasmosis, rubella, cytomegalovirus, and herpes. Syphilis is a sexually transmitted disease (STD) that if left untreated will result in death for about 50% of fetuses during or after the second trimester. Infants who survive may be mentally retarded, blind, or deaf, or all 3.

Toxoplasmosis is an infection with a microorganism (*Toxoplasma gondii*) transmitted to humans from animals, especially cats. It occurs in about 1 or 2 per 1,000 live births. The highest risk to the fetus occurs when the mother contracts the disease in the third trimester, although she may be unaware she is infected. Consequences may include spontaneous abortion, premature birth, SGA infants, and mental retardation.

Rubella (German measles) affects less than 1 per 1,000 live births. If a mother is infected during the first trimester, rubella can cause deafness, heart defects, and cataracts in her child.

Cytomegalovirus (CMV) belongs to the herpes simplex group. CMV infection affects 12–20 of every 1,000 newborns, 5%–10% of whom have significant neurological complications, including mental retardation and hearing problems. An infected fetus may die in utero, or survive with brain damage.

Environmental Hazards

Lead contamination can cause an increased rate of spontaneous abortion, fetal death, and premature birth. Infants who survive are more likely to have poor growth and various neurological difficulties. Pregnant women can be excluded from working with lead; however, exposure is associated with a decreased sperm count in men.

Radiation exposure is a well-known significant risk because it alters fetal cell division and growth. It has been associated with spontaneous abortions, congenital abnormalities, and mental retardation. Fetuses who are exposed are at higher risk for childhood leukemia.

Maternal Illness

Diabetes mellitus, especially Type I insulin-dependent diabetes (IDDM), is characterized by increased levels of blood glucose (hyperglycemia), which crosses the placenta from mother to fetus. Maternal hyperglycemia during the third to sixth week of gestation results in 3–4 times the incidence of congenital anomalies, such as heart defects and hydrocephalus. Later during pregnancy, maternal hyperglycemia stimulates insulin production in the fetus to lower blood glucose levels. This leads to excessive fetal growth, and infants born large for gestational age who are at risk for acute hypoglycemia after birth.

Acquired immunodeficiency syndrome (AIDS) develops in infants whose mothers are positive for HIV. At birth, most infants with prenatal exposure are without symptoms but have positive antibody titers, which indicates transfer of maternal antibodies across the placenta. By 15 months, half of these infants will have shed the maternal antibodies and remain without disease, a phenomenon sometimes referred to as negative seroconversion. Infected infants are more likely to be SGA, experience failure to thrive, and are vulnerable to bacterial and viral infections.

20 Hazards of Prematurity— Part A

A Classification of prematurity

Classification	Gestational Age (wk)	Weight (g)	Characteristics
Borderline premature	36–37	2,500–3,200	Lanugo on skin; fewer creases on feet; genitalia not fully developed; difficulties with breathing, regulating temperature, and feeding; jaundice; 90% chance for healthy survival
Moderately premature	31–35	1,500–2,500	Same as borderline premature only more so; thinner skin; more vascular problems regulating glucose, fluid volume, and red blood cell production; 50% risk for disabilities.
Extremely premature	23–30	400–1,400	No subcutaneous fat beneath paper-thin skin; eyes possibly fused shut; significant respiratory problems; infants <1,000 g have 70% incidence of brain hemorrhage and serious disabilities; those <600 g likely die.

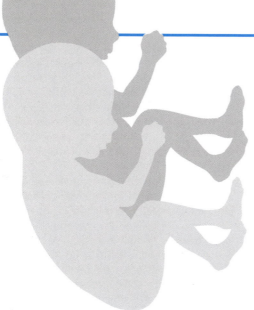

B Risk factors for premature birth

Maternal age <16 and >35 yr
Poor prenatal care
Poor nutrition, anemia
Smoking, substance abuse
Incompetent cervix
Twins, triplets, etc.
Abnormalities of placenta or uterus
Infection, renal disease
Diabetes mellitus
Trauma

Preterm birth is responsible for almost two-thirds of infant mortality. Those who survive are at increased risk for cerebral palsy, mental retardation, and sensory and learning impairments. They also experience more chronic health problems during infancy and childhood. These difficulties have implications for social, educational, and psychological adaptation.

Terms Used to Refer to Prematurity

The average gestational period for the human infant is 40 weeks. The date when the baby's birth is expected is called the estimated date of confinement (EDC). It is calculated by counting backward 3 months from a woman's last menstrual cycle and then adding 7 days. An infant is full term when its birth occurs between 1 week before and 2 weeks after the EDC. The infant weighs 3,100–3,400 g and is about 50 cm long.

According to the World Health Organization, infants are *premature* (or preterm) if born before 37 weeks, regardless of weight. *Low birth weight* (LBW) refers to infants weighing less than 2,500 g at birth, even if they are born at term. *Very low birth weight* (VLBW) refers to infants weighing less than 1,500 g; they are unlikely to be born at term.

Although *premature* and *low birth weight* are often used interchangeably, the determination of prematurity is based on the relationship between weight and gestational age (see **Part A**). *Gestational age* is determined through neurological and physical assessment between 2 and 8 hours after birth. Identifying the point in fetal development at which the infant was born is critical for anticipating problems in the postnatal period. The *corrected age* of a preterm infant is calculated by adding the postnatal age to the gestational age. Thus, an infant born at 30 weeks' gestation 2 weeks ago is considered to be at 32 weeks.

Premature infants are considered *appropriate for their gestational age* (AGA) when their weight at birth is typical for a fetus of the same gestational age. Infants are *small for gestational age* (SGA) when their weight is less than would be expected. Premature infants who weigh more at birth do better. For example, those weighing more than 2,500 g and born after 37 weeks are more likely to survive with good outcomes than those weighing less than 2,000 g born at the same gestational age.

The younger and smaller the infant is, the less mature are the major organ systems essential for sustaining life. The key systems are those that allow the exchange of oxygen (lungs, red blood cells), the absorption of nutrients (gastrointestinal tract), the generation of energy for cell growth (glucose regulation), and autonomic regulation (skin integrity, body temperature, fluid volume, blood pressure, heart rate).

Complications of Prematurity

While there are many complications of prematurity, the most critical organ system is the lungs. Surfactant, which begins to form at about 28 weeks' gestation, allows the alveoli to expand so that oxygen and carbon dioxide can be exchanged. Muscles in the chest wall facilitate expansion of the lungs.

Poor gas exchange at the cellular level has cascading consequences on all major organ systems. The combination of decreased oxygen perfusion, of acid-base imbalances in metabolism and respiration, and of related difficulties with regulation of blood flow can adversely affect the developing brain, the retinas of the eyes, and the intestines, and can also complicate the closure of the patent ductus in the heart. The long-term effects on growth and development vary.

Respiratory distress syndrome (RDS) is related to immature lungs at birth. Because of poor oxygen exchange, the infant is easily fatigued and at risk for pneumonia. Difficulties regulating breathing and heart rate render the infant more vulnerable to stress, such as a cold room or handling. While RDS is usually self-limiting and without long-term effects, it can lead to other problems, especially if an infant requires mechanical ventilation.

Bronchopulmonary dysplasia (BPD) is a chronic lung condition that affects infants who are born prior to 28 weeks' gestation, and who require mechanical ventilation for RDS, which can overexpand and traumatize underdeveloped lungs. BPD develops when infants depend on oxygen for more than 28 days and beyond 36 weeks' gestational age. A family history of asthma is also a factor.

Twenty-five percent of BPD infants die. Survivors experience delays in physical growth and cognitive and language development, although by ages 10–12 years 60% of children with BPD are developmentally normal. Many require nasal oxygen throughout childhood, which limits physical activities and requires special arrangements at school. Children with BPD are at risk for frequent respiratory ailments and asthma.

Periventricular-intraventricular hemorrhage (PIVH) (i.e., bleeding into the ventricles of the brain) is the most common cause of brain damage in premature infants. The incidence is 40% in infants weighing less than 1,500 g, but almost 70% in those weighing less than 1,000 g. Half of PIVHs occur within 24 hours of birth.

The primary cause of PIVH is hypertension. Because autonomic self-regulatory mechanisms are immature, there are fluctuations in blood flow to and blood pressure in the brain. Respiratory distress, infection, traumatic birth, and maternal hypertension during pregnancy can also be factors.

Outcome for the infant depends on the extent and area of hemorrhage, and if there is posthemorrhage hydrocephalus. Half of infants with extensive PIVH die; those who survive are severely disabled. Moderate damage can cause mental retardation and neuromuscular abnormalities. Those with mild PIVH may manifest more subtle difficulties later in childhood, such as learning or emotional disabilities.

21 Hazards of Prematurity— Part B

A Classification of prematurity

Classification	Gestational Age (wk)	Weight (g)	Characteristics
Borderline premature	36–37	2,500–3,200	Lanugo on skin; fewer creases on feet; genitalia not fully developed; difficulties with breathing, regulating temperature, and feeding; jaundice; 90% chance for healthy survival
Moderately premature	31–35	1,500–2,500	Same as borderline premature only more so; thinner skin; more vascular problems regulating glucose, fluid volume, and red blood cell production; 50% risk for disabilities.
Extremely premature	23–30	400–1,400	No subcutaneous fat beneath paper-thin skin; eyes possibly fused shut; significant respiratory problems; infants <1,000 g have 70% incidence of brain hemorrhage and serious disabilities; those <600 g likely die.

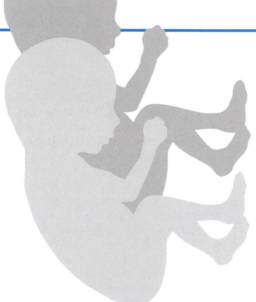

B Risk factors for premature birth

Maternal age <16 and >35 yr
Poor prenatal care
Poor nutrition, anemia
Smoking, substance abuse
Incompetent cervix
Twins, triplets, etc.
Abnormalities of placenta or uterus
Infection, renal disease
Diabetes mellitus
Trauma

Growth and Development

The growth pattern of premature infants is adjusted for corrected age (gestational age plus postnatal age) for 2–3 years after birth. For example, at 6 months after birth, the corrected age of a preterm infant is 4 months; that is, the infant is expected to exhibit characteristics more typical of a 4-month-old baby. LBW babies are still smaller than average at 3 years, even when corrected age is used. By adolescence, most have reached their genetic potential with regard to size.

Head circumference is a good indicator of neuro-developmental outcome. Growth of the head when accompanied by milestones in neuromotor functioning signifies the brain is developing after birth. The critical postnatal period for catch-up growth is 6 weeks to 6 months. The smaller the head is at birth, the less catch-up growth is experienced after birth, regardless of weight and gestational age.

Outcomes have improved. Of infants weighing more than 1,500 g at birth, 90% will demonstrate normal cognitive and motor development by age 2. For infants weighing less than 1,000 g, 50% will be within normal range by age 2.

Implications for Parents and Health Care Providers

Risk factors that contribute to premature birth are noted in **Part B**. Many are preventable. Parenting a premature infant is difficult. Parents must mourn the loss of the healthy child who was not born while anticipating the loss of the premature infant they have. Some parents may avoid becoming emotionally engaged with their infant in the neonatal intensive care unit. At first, they may focus only on hard data, such as blood gas or bilirubin levels. Next, parents may comment on the infant's behavior, such as yawning.

When parents note that the baby is responding to them personally, they begin to claim the child as theirs emotionally. Parents need guidance from nurses and physicians to do this. The behavioral cues of premature infants are harder to read than are those of the typical newborn. Parents may misinterpret cues or overstimulate the baby in an effort to interact with it.

It is important to understand how cues between infants and parents work so that you can facilitate the attachment process. Premature infants are at greater risk for neglect and abuse from overwhelmed parents when they finally go home. Nurses are in a position to intervene early so as to promote optimal outcomes for these tiny babies.

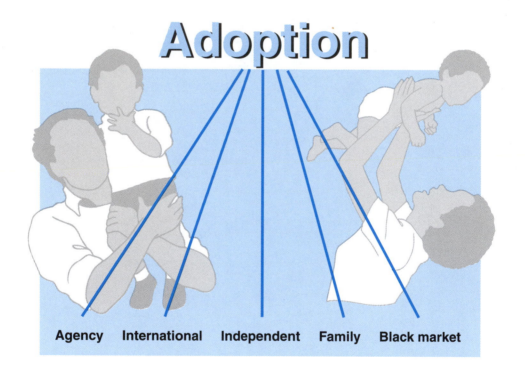

Adoption

Agency   International   Independent   Family   Black market

Couples who remain childless in spite of using assisted reproduction techniques should not feel that they have exhausted all avenues. Adoption (to take a child of other parents voluntarily as one's own) remains an attractive option.

Facts about Adoption

About 2%–4% of children in the United States are adopted. The number of adoptions has been averaging about 120,000 for each of the past several years. Of these, about 50% are adoptions by relatives and 50% between unrelated individuals. About 91% of all adoptions are domestic and 9% are foreign.

In spite of competition among traditional couples, single adults, older adults, and homosexual adults, more children are available for adoption than is commonly thought, but they fall into special categories: older children, minority children, and children with disabilities. While these children are available for immediate adoption, the waiting period for healthy white infants may be years.

Issues Facing Adopting Parents

Couples thinking about adoption should consider carefully several issues they must address at various ages. Given their personalities, interests, and experiences, they will probably be more comfortable with one age group than others.

Infants

Infants are the easiest to adopt because they do not have the experiences older children bring with them. Mother-infant attachment typically proceeds normally.

Preschool Children

Most parents tell children they are adopted when they are around 3 or 4 years old. Parents experience appreciable anxiety during this time, worrying about how and when to tell children. Once children realize they are adopted and understand what that means, the relationship with the adoptive parents inevitably changes, affecting both parents and children. Children, for example, must cope with the idea of being relinquished, not an easy task; parents must accept the idea that their children will want to know more about their biological parents.

School-Age Children

During the 7–12-year period, children with improving cognitive abilities ask certain questions: Who are my parents? Where did I come from? What did my parents look like? Where do they live? Why did they relinquish me? They may well go through a period of grieving for the loss of their family of origin.

Adolescence

With adolescence comes a host of developmental changes. Physical changes, sexual maturation, cognitive advances, and the struggle for identity become important issues for teenagers. Adopted children may be bothered by a lack of any physical similarity to their family. "Genealogical bewilderment" may haunt them, causing them to create a "hereditary ghost," that is, some imaginary figure children create who represents what is good and desirable in their fantasy genetic past. Note that these are possibilities, nothing more.

Closed Adoption

Adoption may take 1 of 2 forms: closed or open. In closed adoptions, biological parents are completely removed from the life of their child; no contact between the parties was allowed before or during the post-placement period. The bonds between birth parent(s) and child were legally and permanently severed; the child's history was sealed by the court. Not only did the law intervene, but also in some extreme cases, women were blindfolded and forced to use earplugs during birth. No chance was taken that any emotional attachments could endure.

Open Adoption

In the 1970s, the concept of closed adoption was challenged on the grounds that both children and biological parents were being needlessly harmed and subjected to unnecessary emotional problems. When a pregnant woman approaches an adoption agency today, she gets what she wants. She can insist that her child be raised by a couple with specific characteristics: nationality, religion, income, number of family members. She can ask to see her child several times a year, perhaps take the youngster on a vacation, and telephone the child frequently. The adoption agency will try to meet these demands.

This process is called open adoption, the sharing of information or contacts between the adoptive and biological parents of an adopted child, before, during, and after placement. Thus, we see a new definition of adoption: the process of accepting the responsibility of raising an individual who has 2 sets of parents.

Implications for Health Care Providers

The positive and negative aspects of adoption have 2 significant implications for health care providers. In a sense, they are 2 sides of the same coin.

- Do not let the fact of a child's adoption lead you to conclude that an adopted child may be more susceptible to problems than any other child. The developmental outcomes of adopted children are generally positive and research to date does not support any other conclusion.
- On the other hand, do not overlook the possibility that there may be problems related to the adoption that could affect recovery.

Directions: For each of the following questions, choose the **one best** answer.

1. What is a gene?

(A) Long strands of deoxyribonucleic acid (DNA)

(B) The sequence in which nucleotide bases are arranged

(C) Multiple combinations of nucleotide bases

(D) The functional units of DNA

2. Skin cells contain

(A) 46 chromosomes.

(B) 23 chromosomes.

(C) 46 autosomes.

(D) 23 sex chromosomes.

3. What process is responsible for genetic variability among human organisms?

(A) Mitosis

(B) Meiosis

(C) Fertilization

(D) Capacitation

4. Where does fertilization occur in the female?

(A) Uterus

(B) Vagina

(C) Fallopian tubes

(D) Ovaries

5. The critical period of organogenesis occurs during

(A) the embryonic period.

(B) the germinal period.

(C) the fetal period.

(D) at the time of conception.

6. Research suggests that insufficient folic acid in the mother's diet may contribute to the failure of the neural tube to close, resulting in spina bifida. At what point in prenatal development does the neural tube close?

(A) 4th week

(B) 8th week

(C) 4th month

(D) 6th month

7. The causes of infertility are

(A) unknown.

(B) male.

(C) female.

(D) male or female.

8. Estimates are that about 1 in _____ American couples are infertile.

(A) 2 or 3

(B) 3 or 4

(C) 5 or 6

(D) 7 or 8

9. A major concern for sperm banks is control of

(A) disease.

(B) donor availability.

(C) confidential information.

(D) technological innovation.

10. For all assisted reproductive technologies (ART), _____ is critical.

(A) location

(B) climate

(C) timing

(D) contingency

11. Genes make up _____% of DNA.

(A) 1

(B) 2

(C) 3

(D) 4

12. The Human Genome Project (HGP) is an attempt to map

(A) all human genes.

(B) cellular materials.

(C) nucleotides.

(D) cell divisions.

13. An example of a genetic disorder is

(A) Down syndrome.

(B) Turner's syndrome.

(C) Klinefelter's syndrome.

(D) sickle-cell anemia.

14. An example of a chromosomal disorder is

(A) spina bifida.

(B) chronic disease syndrome.

(C) phenylketonuria (PKU).

(D) Turner's syndrome.

15. How is prematurity defined?

(A) Infants are premature if born before 37 weeks, regardless of weight.

(B) Infants are premature if they weigh less than 2,500 g at birth, regardless of age.

(C) Infants are premature if they weigh less than 1,500 g and are born before 37 weeks.

(D) Prematurity is based on the relationship between weight and gestational age.

16. The organ system that is most critical to the premature infant's outcome is

(A) the heart.

(B) the lungs.

(C) the brain.

(D) the nervous system.

17. What makes regular use of alcohol during pregnancy a teratogen?

(A) It interferes with fetal cell division and growth throughout pregnancy.

(B) It alters the development of the fetal central nervous system (CNS) during the last trimester.

(C) Women who abuse alcohol are less likely to be well nourished.

(D) All of the above are correct.

18. What is the best-known cause of deafness in newborns?

(A) Cocaine use by mother during pregnancy

(B) Mother's contraction of rubella during the 1st trimester

(C) Mother's exposure to radiation during the last trimester

(D) Mother's exposure to cytomegalovirus (CMV)

19. When a natural mother retains input into the adoption process, this is called _____ adoption.

(A) selected

(B) congruent

(C) accommodated

(D) open

20. Couples considering adoption should think carefully about the _____ of the child.

(A) weight

(B) age

(C) size

(D) cognition

1. The answer is D.

Genes are the functional units of DNA. The DNA molecule consists of chemical compounds called nucleotides, linked together in 2 long chains that coil to form a double helix, which looks like a twisted ladder. The key is the sequence in which the nucleotide bases are arranged along and between the ladder (i.e., on the "sides" and the "rungs"). A *code word* refers to a specific arrangement of 3 bases, and multiple combinations of code words along the DNA strand form genes. Where and how in the longer strand of DNA they start and stop, and whether or not they overlap, depend on the careful placement of specific code words. Genes, sometimes alone, sometimes in combination, contain the coded information that determines particular traits in an individual person.

2. The answer is A.

Skin cells are somatic cells, that is, the cells that make up the major organs and body systems. Genes are arranged in linear order on chromosomes. Somatic cells contain 46 chromosomes arranged in 23 pairs of homologous chromosomes. One of each pair is inherited from each parent. Of the 23 pairs, 22 are autosomes and 1 pair is the sex chromosomes. Autosomes control most body traits, whereas the sex chromosomes determine gender as well as other traits. Females contain 2 X chromosomes: XX. Males contain 1 X and 1 Y chromosome: XY.

3. The answer is B.

Meiosis is the process of cell division by which 1 diploid somatic cell produces 4 haploid gamete cells. First, the 46 chromosomes in the diploid somatic cell replicate, so that each of the 46 chromosomes has a doubled structure. Then, rather than separate into 2 identical cells like in mitosis, the chromosomes literally intertwine. As chromosomes carrying similar genes touch, they exchange genetic material. This exchange is responsible for genetic variability, such as eye color or height. When the original cell divides, it forms 2 cells, each containing 23 chromosomes that are doubled in structure, but in combinations that are different from the original cell.

4. The answer is C.

After the ovum is released by the ovaries, it is carried into the fallopian tubes. Fertilization usually takes place in the outer third of the fallopian tubes, called the ampulla. The mature ovum is fertile for only 24 hours after ovulation. Sperm can survive in the female reproductive tract for 72 hours, but are at peak performance during the first 24 hours. Of the 200–400 million sperm released during ejaculation, only 200 will reach the ampulla in about 4 hours. Only 1 sperm fertilizes an ovum.

5. The answer is A.

Embryo is the name given to the fertilized ovum during the first 8 weeks of prenatal development. The first 2 weeks are also called the germinal period, or the period of the ovum. From 3 to 8 weeks is the critical period of organogenesis, during which all of the major organs develop.

6. The answer is A.

During the 4th week, the heart begins to beat; limb buds are visible; eyes, ears, nerves, and the skeletomuscular and digestive systems begin to form; and the neural tube closes. The embryo is about 0.5 cm long and weighs 0.4 g. Women who are planning to become pregnant should be sure they have adequate amounts of folic acid in their diets.

7. The answer is D.

One of the myths concerning infertility is that it is essentially a female problem. Today, research clearly indicates that the male or the female may be responsible.

8. The answer is C.

These figures testify to the extent of this problem. Research has opened many new possibilities for infertile couples.

9. The answer is A.

Concern about the possibility of disease has caused sperm banks to exercise extreme caution in their screening procedures.

10. The answer is C.

Once detailed information about the reproductive process became available, the timing for the union of sperm and egg was seen as a key element for a successful procedure.

11. The answer is C.

The small amount of genetic material in each cell illustrates the difficulty of the task facing researchers. The rest of the material is referred to as "evolutionary junk."

12. The answer is A.

The HGP is an international effort intended to identify the 50,000–100,000 genes in each cell. These discoveries will lead to many medical breakthroughs.

13. The answer is D.

14. The answer is D.

Knowledge of chromosomal disorders has increased tremendously. Chromosomal disorders seem to be associated with age.

15. The answer is D.

According to the World Health Organization, infants are premature if born before 37 weeks, regardless of weight. Low birth weight (LBW) refers to infants weighing less than 2,500 g at birth, even if they were born at term. Very-low-birth-weight (VLBW) infants weigh less than 1,500 g, and are unlikely to be born at term. Although the terms *premature* and *low birth weight* are often used interchangeably, the determination of prematurity is based on the relationship between weight and gestational age. Gestational age is determined through neurological and physical assessment between 2 and 8 hours after birth. Premature infants are considered appropriate for their gestational age (AGA) when their weight at birth is typical for a fetus of the same gestational age.

16. The answer is B.

While there are many complications of prematurity, the organ system that is most critical to the infant's outcome is the lungs. Surfactant, which begins to form at about 28 weeks' gestation, allows the alveoli to expand so that oxygen and carbon dioxide can be exchanged. Poor gas exchange at the cellular level has cascading consequences on all major organ systems. The combination of decreased oxygen perfusion, of acid-base imbalances in metabolism and respiration, and of related difficulties with regulation of blood flow can adversely affect the developing brain, the retinas of the eyes, and the intestines, and can also complicate the closure of the patent ductus in the heart.

17. The answer is D.

Regular use interferes with fetal cell division and growth throughout pregnancy. During the 3rd trimester in particular, alcohol adversely alters development of the central nervous system (CNS) and brain. Alcohol constitutes empty calories; that is, it has no nutritional value but contributes to weight gain. Women who abuse alcohol during pregnancy are less likely to eat well and to seek regular prenatal care. Fetal alcohol syndrome is found in about 40% of infants born to alcoholics.

18. The answer is B.

Rubella (German measles) affects less than 1 per 1,000 live births. If a mother is infected during the 1st trimester, rubella can cause deafness, heart defects, and cataracts in her child.

19. The answer is D.

Since the number of children available for adoption are far less than the demand, a woman today may exercise considerable control over the adoption process.

20. The answer is B.

In opting for adoption, parents should be aware of a child's age in light of their own compatibility with a particular age group. Other characteristics, such as weight, for example, usually lack the same impact on a relationship as age.

PART III
Infancy

23 Neonatal Assessment

A Apgar scoring

Sign	0	1	2
Heart rate	Absent	Slow (< 100)	>100
Respiratory effort	Absent	Slow, irregular	Good cry
Muscle tone	Flaccid	Some flexion of extremities	Active motion
Reflex irritability	No response	Cry	Vigorous cry
Color[a]	Blue, pale	Body pink, extremities blue	Completely pink

[a] Blue indicates cyanosis, i.e., poor perfusion of oxygenated blood; pink indicates the skin is well perfused. The colors are not intended to indicate racial characteristics.

B Normal vital signs in newborns (0–28 days)

Heart rate	Respirations	Blood Pressure	Temperature	Neuromuscular
120–140/min apical	30–60/min abdominal breathing	65/41 mm Hg in arm or calf, increases with crying	36.5–37.0°C axillary, increases with crying	Extremities flexed, can extend; arms rest on chest; when prone, holds head in line with back, turns it to side

C Neonatal Behaviors in Brazelton Neonatal Assessment Scale

Habituation: baby attends to novel stimuli, gets used to it, inhibits attention

Orientation: baby is alert and attending to stimuli

Motor performance: movement and tone

Range of state: arousal level

Regulation of state: baby responds when aroused

Autonomic stability: homeostatic regulation

Reflexes: inborn neuromotor behaviors

Physical Changes

The transition from uterine to extrauterine life happens in moments. The initial breath is probably triggered by changes in pressure on the thorax during birth. Fluid is squeezed from the lungs and replaced by a rush of air. Within 1 minute, the brain stem picks up signals about the rise and fall of arterial oxygen and carbon dioxide, triggering a gasping breath and crying. The lungs clear, promoting the conversion from fetal to infant heart-lung circulation. Sensory changes such as air temperature, noise, and light also contribute to the first breath.

Apgar scores are used as a rough assessment of immediate adjustment to extrauterine life. Heart rate, respirations, muscle tone, reflexes, and skin color are assessed at 1 and 5 minutes after birth, with each given a score of 0, 1, or 2 (see **Part A**). Total scores lower than

3 indicate severe distress. Scores of 4–6 signify moderate difficulty, and scores of 7–10 indicate no difficulty adapting to extrauterine life. Apgar scores are affected by prematurity and maternal medication, and are not indicative of the presence or absence of neurological or physical abnormalities. **Part B** cites normal vital signs in newborns.

During the first 24 hours, healthy newborns undergo predictable changes in physiological and behavioral processes. The *first period of reactivity* covers the initial 6–8 hours. For the first 30 minutes, infants are highly active. They cry, suck their fists, and pass meconium and urine. Mucus secretions, heart rate, and respirations increase. Then they become attentive to their surroundings, with eyes open, and will nurse vigorously. During the second stage, which lasts 2–4 hours, heart and respiratory rates and body temperature decrease as infants become calm. They sleep deeply, blocking out stimuli. The *second period of reactivity* follows. Infants are alert and responsive, providing an optimal situation for parents and newborns to interact. Heart rate and respirations increase again, and then stabilize.

The *New Ballard Scale* is used to determine gestational age in infants who are born prematurely or who are small or large for their apparent gestational age (Ballard et al., 1991). Maturity is rated on a scale from −1 to +5 in 13 areas, such as flexion of extremities, quality of skin, creases on the sole of the feet, and development of eyes, ears, and genitals. Total scores range from −10 (20 weeks' gestation, extremely premature) to +50 (44 weeks' gestation, postmature). The combination of accurate gestational age and birth weight are good predictors of perinatal morbidity and mortality.

Behavioral Assessment

Newborns arrive preadapted to interact with the physical and social environment. Parents often ask if their baby can see them. The answer is yes. Although visual acuity at birth is between 20/100 and 20/400, newborns can see and fixate on objects within 20 cm of the center of their bodies. They can see their parents' faces clearly while being held or bathed. Babies have an inborn preference for looking at complex patterns rather than solid fields. They prefer light and dark patterns over color, and visually follow a moving object.

Human faces fit these criteria. Babies gaze at their parents with great interest, a behavior that endears them to parents and enhances survival. Newborns also prefer the sound of human voices, and at birth will turn their heads toward any sound to locate it. At 3 days, newborns discriminate their mother's voice from that of other women. At 5 days, they use their sense of smell to identify their mother's breast milk.

Newborn behavior has 4 characteristics. (1) Inborn physiological mechanisms, such as reflexes, enhance *survival*. (2) Newborns *organize their behavior* in response to stimuli (e.g., turning their heads in response to a sound). (3) They *respond selectively* to certain stimuli (e.g., patterns of light and dark). (4) Newborns demonstrate *contingency-seeking* behavior; that is, they look for predictability in the environment) for events that go together. Thus we refer to the preadapted neonate as a *competent infant*.

The *Brazelton Neonatal Behavioral Assessment Scale* (BNBAS), developed by T. Berry Brazelton, is based on these characteristics. It is designed to assess 28 newborn behaviors, clustered in 7 areas (see **Part C**). A key factor is the newborn's state of consciousness at the time of the assessment. The BNBAS identifies 6 states along a continuum from deep sleep to active and alert (Brazelton & Nugent, 1996).

Infants are not easily aroused from *deep sleep*, during which time their breathing is regular. During *light sleep*, breathing is irregular and infants can be awakened by a noise. *Drowsy* infants have their eyes open and are aroused by stimuli; breathing is irregular, and they squirm. *Quiet alert* infants are attentive. Their eyes are open, they orient to stimuli, and may coo or smile. Breathing is regular. *Active alert* infants are fussy and restless. They respond to stimuli, but may not attend for long. *Crying* ranges from whimpering to howling. Stimuli are shut out.

The best time to perform the BNBAS is when infants are quiet and alert. This is also the optimal time for parent-infant interaction. During the BNBAS, a trained evaluator observes how the infant responds to various stimuli, such as handling, sounds, light, and so on. The evaluator looks for discrete responses to stimuli, and how the infant organizes its state. For example, can a fussy baby reorganize itself to become quiet and alert in response to the evaluator's voice and touch? The BNBAS shows parents what their baby is capable of and how it responds to voices, touch, and faces.

Self-regulation and Infant Learning

Evidence of infant learning is based on the inborn tendency to seek out contingencies and to build on reflexes. Volitional control over the sucking reflex increases in the first few weeks of life. In a classic experiment, DeCasper and Fifer (1980) demonstrated that infants can learn to adjust their rate of sucking, using the mother's voice as a reward. When they sucked at a fast pace, a tape of the mother's voice was played. They also learned a reverse contingency wherein the tape played only when they sucked slowly.

Thus we see that infants begin to regulate their own behavior in response to environmental stimuli. Infants have the inborn capacity to self-quiet, to reorganize, and to pay attention to their surroundings. They learn to do so of their own volition in the context of sensitive caretaking by parents. Distressed infants who are firmly but gently held, who hear a soothing voice and smell a familiar smell, and who can predict that a cry will get a caring response learn to use parents as a resource to help them regulate their own behavioral state. That is the beginning of trust.

24 Reflexes

A Simple reflex arc

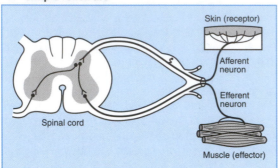

B Babinski reflex

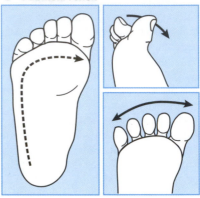

C Reflexes that change or disappear with neurological maturity

Reflex	Stimulus and Response	Comments
Babinski	Stroke the sole of foot as shown in Part B. Toes fan out and extend; big toe dorsiflexes.	Gone by 1 year of age. With maturity, toes flex.
Tonic neck	Turn infants head to one side while lying on back. Arm and leg on that side extend; arm and leg on the opposite side flex (looks like a fencer's stance).	Disappears after 3–4 months. Response becomes symmetric.
Stepping	Hold infant upright with feet lightly touching surface. Feet step rhythmically in place. Term infants step on the soles of feet; preterm infants step with toes.	Present for 3–4 weeks after term, then fades.
Plantar	Apply pressure with finger against ball of foot. All toes plantar flex, grasping the finger.	Lessens by 8 months; gone by 1 year.
Startle	Stimulus is a loud noise. Response is similar to Moro reflex. Arms at first flail out, then pull in; fists clench.	Present for 3–4 weeks.
Crawling	Place newborn on abdomen. Infant makes crawling movement with arms and legs.	Gone by about 6 weeks.

D Permanent reflexes designed to protect against harm

Reflex	Stimulus and Response	Comments
Blinking	Flash light in eyes or brush against eyelashes. Eyes close.	Protects eyes.
Gag	Touch back of throat (pharynx). Person gags as throat closes.	Prevents objects in mouth from entering trachea.
Withdrawal	Prick sole of foot with a pin. Person pulls foot away.	Protective reflex. With repeated pricks, response fades.

Reflexes are involuntary stimulus-response behaviors of the human nervous system. The sequence of neural events that gives rise to reflexive behaviors is called the *reflex arc*: (1) A receptor organ (skin, eye, mouth) receives a stimulus from the external environment (hot touch, bright light, sour taste); (2) information about the stimulus is transmitted along a sensory, that is afferent, neuron in the peripheral nervous system (PNS) to (3) a specialized region of the CNS where the information is integrated and synapse occurs; (4) the CNS relays the synaptic impulse to a motor neuron in the PNS, which transmits it to (5) an effector organ (muscles, glands) that produces the observable behavior called a *reflex*. The conduction of all of this information is facilitated by the *myelin sheaths* that insulate the nerve cells along the reflex arc (see **Part A**).

The specialized regions that give rise to reflexes are found in the more primitive areas of the CNS, such as the spinal cord, brain stem, and cerebellum. In terms of evolutionary biology, reflexes are built-in mechanisms that sustain life and allow humans to react to threat without thinking. As reviewed in Chapter 27, the CNS is not fully developed at birth, and continues to grow, reorganize, and mature. For example, myelination of the nerve cells in the cerebellum, which coordinates sensory-motor information, continues for several years.

Because their nervous systems are maturing, infants exhibit reflexive behaviors that are different from those found in older children and adults. Infant reflexes are interesting for several reasons. Some are adaptive behaviors arising from the primitive CNS, which develops early in utero and infancy, before the higher regions of the cortex which are responsible for thinking and volitional behavior. These reflexes are adaptive because the primitive CNS also developed early in the evolution of our history as human primates, and have helped to ensure the survival of our young. Some adaptive infant reflexes are building blocks for voluntary motor behaviors that develop with experience and with maturity of the cortical regions of the brain. Thus, reflexes can also provide a window into neurological development because they should change as the nervous system matures (see **Parts B** and **C**). Finally, some reflexes are permanent throughout life, designed to protect us from potential harm (see **Part D**).

Reflexes That Are Adaptive Behaviors

Rooting
Stroke an infant's cheek, and the head turns to that side, the mouth opens, and the infant attempts to suck your finger. This reflex is adaptive because it facilitates feeding. The touch of the breast against the infant's cheek elicits this response. Rooting disappears by 4 months.

Sucking
Put your finger or a nipple into the infant's mouth. The infant begins sucking rhythmically. This reflex is adap-

tive because it is essential for feeding. Premature infants may not suck, which can threaten their survival. Reflexive sucking disappears by age 2 months as infants gain control over a "burst-pause" pattern in their sucking. They suck vigorously in short bursts, then pause, breaking the tension at the nipple. As the mouth releases, the infant appears to smile. The mother smiles, and speaks to her infant. The infant attends to this interesting and cozy stimulus, focusing the eyes, cooing. In this way, reflexive sucking is a building block for voluntary mother-child interactions.

Moro
Hold an infant horizontally on its back above a dressing table. Suddenly, lower the infant about 6 inches and stop abruptly, simulating a free fall. Or, with the infant lying on the back, raise the head slightly and then release it suddenly, again allowing the infant to feel the force of gravity. In either case, the infant extends the arms, throws back the head, and spreads the fingers. Then the infant brings the arms back to the center of the body with hands clenched, and the spine and legs extended. This reflex is adaptive when you consider our evolutionary roots as primates. The infant feels like it is falling, displays alarm to the mother, and then tries to grab on for safety, a mechanism that would serve infant monkeys in tall treetops well. The Moro reflex weakens by 5 months, and disappears by 8 months.

Grasping
Place an object in the palm of an infant's hand. The infant will curl the fingers around the object strongly enough to hold the infant's weight. Grasping on for dear life is adaptive behavior in young primates. It is also a building block for the complex skill of grabbing and letting go that evolves over the first year. By 3–4 months, the grasping reflex declines, and infants will involuntarily let go of objects placed in their palm. By 4 months, they voluntarily grasp an object by closing their whole palm over it, but cannot let go. By 5 months, they reach and grasp what is in their line of view, but do not have full control over letting go. By 6 months, infants deliberately reach, and grab with their whole hand and thumb like a mitten. Once sitting up at 6–8 months, infants transfer objects from hand to hand across the midline of their bodies, and release objects at will. By 9–12 months, they control the individual movements of the thumb and forefinger to use a pincer-like grasp to pick up finger foods.

Grasping is a good example of how development evolves. It begins with a behavior that is global and diffuse (grasp reflex), becomes more differentiated (palmar grasp evolves into the mitten grasp in which the thumb is separate), and is finally hierarchically integrated. Sitting in a high chair using the pincer grasp to pick up food requires the integrated development of hand-eye coordination, spatial relationships, chewing, and swallowing.

25 Growth and Development I

A Height and Weight Measurements: Boys

Age (mos)	Height by percentiles (cm)			Weight by percentiles (kg)		
	5th	50th	95th	5th	50th	95th
Birth	46.4	50.5	54.4	2.54	3.27	4.15
3	56.7	61.1	65.4	4.43	5.98	7.37
6	63.4	67.8	72.3	6.20	7.85	9.46
9	68.0	72.3	77.1	7.52	9.18	10.93
12	71.7	76.1	81.2	8.43	10.15	11.99
18	77.5	82.4	88.1	9.59	11.47	13.44
24	82.5	86.8	94.4	10.49	12.34	15.50

B Height and Weight Measurements: Girls

Age (mos)	Height by percentiles (cm)			Weight by percentiles (kg)		
	5th	50th	95th	5th	50th	95th
Birth	45.4	49.9	52.9	2.36	3.23	3.81
3	55.4	59.5	63.4	4.18	5.40	6.74
6	61.8	65.9	70.2	5.79	7.21	8.73
9	66.1	70.4	75.0	7.00	8.56	10.17
12	69.8	74.3	79.1	7.84	9.53	11.24
18	76.0	80.9	86.1	8.92	10.82	12.76
24	81.6	86.8	93.6	9.95	11.8	14.15

During the first year, infants grow rapidly. During the second year, the rate of physical growth slows, and there are significant gains in cognition and language. On average, boys are bigger than girls. The data in **Parts A** and **B** are based on national averages of all American-born children. Separate tables for different racial and ethnic groups are available from the National Center for Health Statistics. Tables developed for children who were born prematurely or who have Down syndrome are often used by pediatricians and nurses.

Height, Weight, and Head Circumference: First Year

The average American newborn weighs 3.27 kg. By the second day of life, newborns lose 5%–10% of their birth weight, but steadily regain it by 14 days. This loss is not a problem for healthy babies who are born with a reserve of fat that helps them get through the first few days of life until their mother's breast milk supply is established. Infants then gain 680 g each month until 5–6 months, when their birth weight doubles. Birth weight triples by the end of the first year, to about 10 kg.

By 1 year, birth height has increased by 50%. During the first 6 months, height increases 2.5 cm a month from the average 50 cm at birth, and then slows during the second half of the first year. Most of this growth is in the trunk, not the legs. A typical 1-year-old is around 76 cm tall. Birth height doubles by 4 years.

Head circumference increases during the first year from 33.0 to 35.5 cm to about 46.5 cm, an increase of almost 33%. The weight of the brain has more than doubled. Growth of the head is indicative of brain maturation, which is best seen in the extraordinary motor and sensory achievements of the first year (see Chapter 24).

Height, Weight, and Head Circumference: Second Year

The rate of growth slows during the toddler years. At age 2 years, the average toddler weighs about 12 kg and is 86.8 cm tall. During the second year, most of the growth in height is in the legs and not the trunk. Children's adult height can be estimated by doubling their height at age 2. Head circumference increases by only 2.5 cm during the second year to about 49 cm. It takes another 16 years to add 7 cm to reach adult size.

Nutrition

Human breast milk is the best diet for infants during the first 6 months of life. Milk from a well-nourished mother contains all of the nutrients essential for sustaining newborn life and promoting infant growth. The digestive tracts of young infants are not fully mature, and cannot adequately extract nutrients from fruits, vegetables, and meats, even in pureed form. Cow's milk should not be used because it is poorly digested and causes cramping. Breast milk also contains maternal antibodies against common illnesses that help to protect infants while their immune systems are still developing. Commercial infant formulas are an acceptable substitute if a mother does not wish to breast-feed.

Feeding, especially breast-feeding, contributes to development in other ways. Sucking is an inborn reflex, but feeding is a learned behavior that contributes to self-regulation in infants and sensitive responding in mothers. Mother and infant learn to coordinate supply and demand of milk. This give-and-take requires that mothers learn to read infant signals of hunger, fatigue, distress, and satisfaction. As infants learn to regulate the flow of milk, they also learn to organize their own behavior. Feeding, especially at the breast, helps them to calm down and focus. An attentive infant in the arms of a responsive mother is ready to interact with her, to focus its eyes on her face and listen to her voice.

These types of interactions, whether with mothers, fathers, or other responsive caretakers, are the foundation of trust. Trust versus mistrust is the first of Erikson's stages of the human life cycle. Viewed in evolutionary terms, eating is a fundamental social event that bonds family members together.

Solid foods in pureed form can be introduced at about 5–6 months, when teeth begin to appear and infants can sit up with support. Finger foods can be introduced toward the end of the first year. By 1 year, infant digestive tracts can handle the usual family diet.

Toddlers develop strong likes and dislikes in foods. They prefer to feed themselves or to just play with the food. Not only is this messy, but also parents worry that toddlers are not adequately nourished. As physical growth slows and gross-motor skills improve, busy toddlers typically have decreased appetites. They benefit from frequent snacking throughout the day.

Sleep

The wake-sleep cycles of infants are referred to as *states* (see Chapter 22), which form a continuum of arousal. Newborns are in deep sleep (i.e., they are not easily aroused) for 4–5 hours a day at intervals of 10–20 minutes. Light sleep takes up 12–15 hours of their day, with longer intervals of 20–45 minutes. Breast-fed infants usually sleep for somewhat shorter periods of time because they eat more often.

Infants develop a nocturnal sleep pattern through a combination of physical and neurological maturity and self-regulation in response to parents' efforts to promote predictable feeding, waking, and sleeping habits. By 3–4 months, infants sleep about 9 hours at night and nap about 3 times a day for an hour or so at a time. By the end of the first year, babies nap twice a day, and then only once a day by 18 months. They extend their nighttime sleep to 11–12 hours.

Failure to Thrive (FTT)

FTT is usually diagnosed during the first year of life. Weight falls below the third to fifth percentile, there is deviation from the growth curve, and the characteristic posturing and interactive behaviors of infancy may be absent. There is often a history of feeding and sleeping disturbances and irritability. There are two types of FTT: organic and nonorganic. Organic FTT has physical causes (e.g., digestive, endocrine, or enzyme disorders). Infants who have neurological deficits or are fatigued due to heart defects or infections may not feed well. Nonorganic FTT is usually caused by psychosocial factors (e.g., poverty, lack of knowledge about infant nutrition, inconsistent and poor quality of infant care, and disturbances in maternal-child attachment).

26 Growth and Development II

Sensory/perceptual and motor milestones

Age	Gross Motor	Fine Motor	Sensory/Perceptual
1–3 mo	When prone, lifts head a little, finally to 45 degrees Head lag when pulled to sit lessens	Grasp reflex strong, then gone by 3 mo Hands begin to open, hold rattle, pull at blankets	Visual acuity 20/100 at birth When supine, visually follows light to midline, to side, to 180 degrees
4–6 mo	When prone, raises head and shoulders 90 degrees Rolls back to side, belly to back, back to front Sits with support	Plays with hands, toes Inspects clothing, blankets Grasps objects with both hands, e.g., bottle Brings objects to mouth	Has binocular vision Early hand-eye coordination Visually follows an object when it is dropped Localizes sounds by looking
7–9 mo	Sits alone Sits to play Pulls to stand, falls to sit Creeps, starts to crawl	Transfers objects hand to hand, bangs them on table Grabs and releases objects Early pincer grasp	Aware of depth and spatial relationships Responds to own name Has taste preferences
10–12 mo	Moves from prone to sitting Stands holding furniture, cruises, may walk Can sit down from standing	Eats using fingers Good pincer grasp Grasps spoon by handle Flips pages in book	Drops objects just to watch them fall Fascinated by "in" and "out"
13–15 mo	Walks alone Creeps upstairs	Handedness is apparent Throws things down Scribbles, uses cup	Intense interest in pictures Identifies forms, e.g., circle Good binocular vision
16–18 mo	Runs but falls Walks upstairs with help Jumps in place	Builds tower of 3–4 cubes Manages with spoon Tries to imitate your scribble	
By 24 mo	Walks upstairs 2 feet at a time, runs well Bends down to pick things up without falling	Turns pages in book to "read" Turns doorknobs, unscrews lids	Accommodation of eyes well developed Discriminates pictures of objects

Gross-motor development refers to the infant's ability to control large muscle groups (e.g., lifting the head, crawling). Fine-motor development refers to manual skills (e.g., reaching, grasping). Motor development is closely tied to sensory development. For example, reaching and grasping require hand-eye coordination.

Sequencing of motor development proceeds in a cephalocaudal direction, that is, from head to toe. The brain matures in such a way that babies can control their heads, shoulders, and arms before they can control their legs. Children who persistently lag behind in meeting milestones (see **Table**) need to be assessed for evidence of developmental delay.

Gross-Motor Development

Head control is a good indicator of brain maturation. Newborns turn their head to the side to free their nose when lying on their abdomen on a flat surface. But they cannot lift their head until they are 6 weeks old, and then do so briefly. By 3–4 months, they raise their head, shoulders, and upper body while supporting themselves on their forearms. When newborns are pulled to sit, their head falls back. Head lag decreases and infants have steady head control by 5–6 months, when they can sit with support.

Infants begin purposely *rolling* from their back to one side at 4 months. As they begin raising their upper body from a flat surface by pushing up with their arms, they learn to flip from their abdomen to their back. Rolling from back to front is accomplished by 6 months.

During the first 2 months, infants need to be in a position of full body support. By 5 months, they can *sit up* with back support, and by 7 months they sit alone, leaning forward onto their hands. Infants can sit alone securely by 8 months, with their hands free to manipulate objects.

While many infants begin to propel themselves backward by pushing with their arms when they are lying prone, *true locomotion* implies bearing body weight. Pushing backward gives way to crawling forward with their abdomen still on the floor at about 7 months. Once babies begin creeping on all 4 limbs by 9 months, they are very mobile.

Infants' legs can hold their weight by 8 months, but they do not pull themselves into a standing position holding onto furniture until 9 months. At first, they sit down by letting go and falling. By 1 year, they ease themselves down. It takes several more months to stand, bend down, and sit without holding on. Pulling to stand gives way to cruising by 10–12 months. First steps typically follow around 13–15 months.

This sequence is a generalization of infant development. Some infants never crawl, and are quite content to sit and play. One day, they cruise and the next day they walk. Others are barely walking when suddenly they are climbing stairs. Toddlers have the physical ability and the motivation to be on the move, but lack the judgment their newfound abilities require.

Fine-Motor Development

As noted in Chapter 24, the ability to use the hands is built on a primitive grasping reflex. At birth, infants close their entire hand around an object (e.g., a parent's finger) placed in their palm. As the brain matures, the reflex fades (by 3 months) and infants begin to control grasping and letting go.

Over time, they hold something (e.g., a rattle) that is given to them (3 months), hold a bottle with 2 hands (4 months), grasp using the whole hand (5 months), begin to release objects (6 months), transfer hand to hand (7 months), and finally grasp and release at will (8 months). At the same time, their grip becomes more refined, from using the whole hand, to isolating the thumb (6–8 months), and finally developing a pincer grasp, using the thumb and forefinger (9–10 months).

Sensory/Perceptual Development

Infants are born ready to process visual and auditory information, movement of objects, and the spatial relationship between their body and the physical space they inhabit. Fine- and gross-motor development is closely integrated with changes in perceptual development. They cannot reach and grab something if they cannot judge how far away it is.

At birth, visual acuity is about 20/100 and steadily improves. Objects within close range, like the mother's face, are perfectly clear. A preference for patterns is evident within hours after birth. Infants do not discern color until 2 months. Patterns that are somewhat complex and that have moving parts are of greatest interest, especially the human face. Infants recognize pictures of their mother by 3 months, and prefer pictures of children over adults. They discriminate their mother's voice from others at 3 days, having heard it since the fourth month of gestation.

Binocular vision, which means that the different images taken in by 2 eyes are integrated into 1 picture in the brain, begins to develop at 6 weeks and is well established by 4 months. Binocular vision is related to hand-eye coordination, which first appears at 4 months as infants are learning to grasp voluntarily. Hand-eye coordination continues to mature into childhood.

Depth perception develops, not coincidentally, when infants need to appreciate near and far, that is, when they start to creep, crawl, and cruise during the second half of the first year. About this time, infants become fascinated by falling objects, dropping spoons from their high chair just to watch them fall. In a classic study involving a "visual cliff" (Gibson and Walk, 1960), infants are placed on a level glass surface. On the shallow side, they can see the "floor," a black-and-white tile pattern, a few inches below them. On the deep side, the "floor" is 2 feet or so below them. Infants who appreciate depth will not crawl from the shallow to the deep side.

27 Brain Development

The timing of brain development

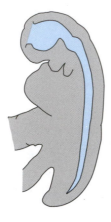

Neural induction
(begins during the 3rd week)

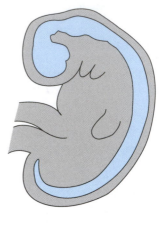

Neural tube
(closes by the end of the 4th week)

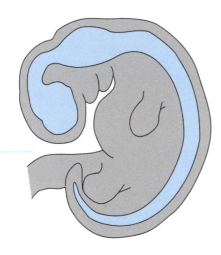

Cell proliferation
(begins during the 5th week)

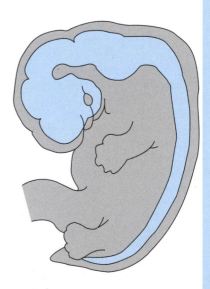

Cell migration
(begins during the 7th week)

Any aspect of development—physical, emotional, cognitive, psychosocial—depends on the intricacy of the brain for its optimal development. In spite of today's sophisticated technology, just how many neurons develop in the course of a lifetime is not precisely known. An estimate is anywhere from 100 billion to 200 billion. For example, the appearance of new cognitive abilities is correlated with rapid brain growth, both of which are major features of infancy.

Beginnings of Brain Development

The beginning of brain development (about the third prenatal week) lies in a process called *neural induction* when a chemical signal from the mesoderm to the ectoderm triggers the onset of nervous system development. Nerve cells proliferate rapidly in the *neural tube*, but quickly leave this area and commence a sometimes lengthy, tortuous, even perilous journey to the region of the brain where they will become functional. This phase, called *cell migration*, begins during the seventh prenatal week. During their passage, the nerve cells may double back, twist, and turn—some will even die. In their migration the nerve cells continue to grow and develop and acquire the neuronal shape most of us are familiar with. Those destined for survival reach their point of destination and become functional. Each of these nerve cells, now called *neurons*, will make connections (called *synapses*) with as many as 10,000 to 200,000 other neurons.

Continuation of Brain Development

Nervous system development begins during the embryonic period when neurons reproduce at a rapid rate. During infancy, connections among the neurons continue to increase, perhaps into the thousands for each of the billions of neurons. This amazing complexity provides the biological basis for cognitive development. Estimates are that the baby's brain at birth is about one-fourth of its adult size. It is about 50% of its adult weight at 6 months, 60% at 1 year, 75% at 2½ years, 90% at 6 years, and 95% at 10 years. In other words, while the brain takes 2½ years to grow to 75% of its adult weight, in another 3½ years growth increases only by 15%.

In the first 2 years following birth, brain development follows a definite pattern; that is, different parts develop at different rates:

- The motor area is the most advanced (for survival purposes) followed in descending order by the sensory area, the visual area, and the auditory area.
- The association areas—the areas devoted to thinking and reasoning—are the slowest to develop.
- By the age of 2 years, growth in the sensory area slows and the association area shows signs of rapid development.

Each of the brain's 4 lobes (frontal, parietal, temporal, and occipital) exercises specialized functions. For example, the frontal lobe contains the motor area for control of all the skeletal muscles, the parietal lobe seems to be the controlling center for the body's sense areas, the temporal lobe manages auditory functions, and the occipital lobe analyzes visual information. Brain structures for thinking are diffused throughout the cortical area, which makes considerable sense when you think about the thought processes involved in answering a question: You listen to the question (auditory area), you respond by speaking (motor area), and you search your memory (association area) (Dacey and Travers, 1999).

Brain Lateralization

The stroke unit of any hospital offers powerful evidence of hemispheric brain damage. A stroke implies a stoppage of blood flow to a certain area of the brain, resulting in damage to that spot. Usually only 1 side of the brain is affected and stroke victims are typically paralyzed on either the left or the right side of the body. In patients with right-side paralysis, the stroke damaged the left side of the brain; in patients with left-side paralysis, the damage was done to the right side of the brain.

It was not until the latter part of the 19th century, however, that right-side paralysis plus loss of speech was linked to damage to the left hemisphere. It took even longer to recognize the contributions that the right hemisphere makes to human functioning (Springer and Deutsch, 1998).

Language is an excellent example of lateralization because language entails the combining of discrete elements—letters, syllables, words. In about 95%–99% of right-handed people and about 70% of left-handed people, language is lateralized to the left side of the brain. Yet researchers cannot be absolutely sure that the right hemisphere is totally inactive in language usage. Blood flow studies suggest that during language processing, considerable blood flows to the right hemisphere as well (Temple, 1993).

Implications for Health Care Providers

As a health care provider, remember that brain development is not complete at birth. To ensure continued growth, the brain requires appropriate stimulation from the environment. In your work with infants, observe how the parents talk to their child. This interaction is a major stimulator during these early years and has a dynamic, effective influence on nervous system development. Urge parents to vary stimulation—auditory, visual, tactile—in their infant's surroundings, thus providing a rich texture for brain development.

28 Cognitive Development

A Development of object permanence according to Piaget

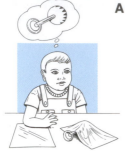

Substages 1 and 2 (0–4 mo):
Infants do not search for an object if it disappears from view.

Substage 3 (4–8 mo):
Babies will search for an object partially hidden under a cloth; that is, they use visual cues to call up the picture of the object.

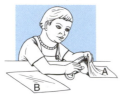

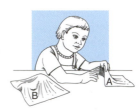

Substage 4 (8–12 mo): Stage 4 error: A-not-B Show baby you are hiding toy under a cloth (A), baby will search for it under the cloth. Do this a few times. Show baby you are hiding it under a second cloth (B) nearby, babies will still search under the first cloth (A).

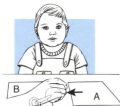

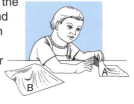

Substage 5 (12–18 mo): Babies no longer make the substage 4 error, and will search under the second cloth where they saw you hide the toy. Now, reach under the first cloth (A), conceal the toy in your hand, and have the baby watch you move it under the second cloth (B). The baby will search under A; he couldn't follow the toy to B in his mind because he didn't see it for real.

Substage 6 (18–24 mo): Objects are known to exist out of sight. The baby can't see a ball as it rolls under a chair, but follows its trajectory in his or her mind and searches where it should end up.

B Habituation event

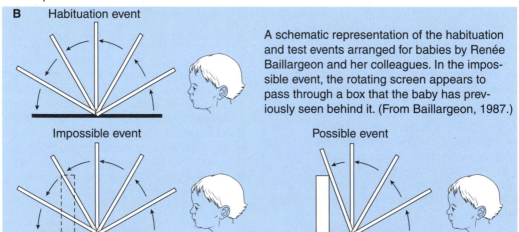

A schematic representation of the habituation and test events arranged for babies by Renée Baillargeon and her colleagues. In the impossible event, the rotating screen appears to pass through a box that the baby has previously seen behind it. (From Baillargeon, 1987.)

Impossible event

Possible event

The competent infant is born ready to learn, and learning promotes development of the brain. Infants demonstrate learning by organizing their behavior in response to stimuli. To make sense of stimuli, they coordinate information using their sensory, physical, mental, and perceptual abilities. Newborns do this differently than do infants 6 or 12 months old because these abilities develop and become better coordinated with maturity and experience.

Piaget's Sensorimotor Period

By "sensorimotor," Piaget meant that mental life begins with infants' ability to interact with the physical environment using their bodies. Physical actions are joined by a growing awareness of how behavior affects the environment. There are 4 accomplishments in this period: (1) spatial relationships—in and out, up and down, near and far; (2) time—before and after; (3) causality—cause and effect, one event leads to another; and (4) object permanence—objects exist when out of sight (see **Part A**). There are 6 substages of the sensorimotor period:

Substage 1 (0–6 weeks [neonate]): reflexes. Infants' behavior is based on inborn reflexes, such as sucking, rooting, and grasping.

Substage 2 (1–4 months): primary circular reactions. As infants gain more motor control over their own bodies (primary), they repeat movements (circular) just for the sake of doing so (e.g., sucking their fingers, kicking their legs).

Substage 3 (4–8 months): secondary circular reactions. Infants use their bodies to act on the physical environment (secondary), repeating actions (circular) because they produce a desired effect. Infants realize they can make things happen. Examples include shaking a rattle, hitting a hanging toy to make it swing, and patting and squeezing toys.

Substage 4 (8–12 months): coordination of secondary circular reactions. One action is performed as a means of achieving another action. Babies can think 1 step ahead, which is highly adaptive when they can crawl or cruise. An example is pushing a toy out of the way to get to the light socket.

Substage 5 (12–18 months): tertiary circular reactions. Actions are performed to learn about the possible relationship between different actions and objects. The busy toddler is experimenting with effects. For example, a ball, a block, and a cat bounce differently when you drop them down the stairs. Tossing the same toy with different amounts of force also produces different effects.

Substage 6 (18–24 months): beginning of representational thought. Representational thought is the ability to picture objects, places, and events in the mind. It is related to language development. Toddlers think about actions and their consequences based on previous experience, and adjust their behavior accordingly. For example, toddlers may place their cup away from the edge of the table so that it won't fall.

Piaget's theory has been challenged by others who found that infants develop some cognitive abilities earlier than he thought. His theory was built on observations of children, especially his own, whereas others tested infants under more structured research conditions. The type of task that is used to measure what infants know shapes the findings.

Other Research

One way to study infant cognition is to rely on infants' inborn tendency to pay attention to novel stimuli and then to habituate to it; that is, they lose interest when it is no longer new and renew interest when the stimuli changes again. Studies are also based on contingency-seeking behavior; that is, infants look for events that go together. When infants respond to events based on previous experience, it implies they can organize, store, and retrieve their experience of events cognitively.

Memory

At 3 months, infants can remember a contingency for up to a week, and as much as a month later if given a visual cue. For example, if taught to make a mobile move by kicking 1 leg, which is attached to the mobile by a ribbon, infants will kick again a week later. A month later, if the babies are shown the mobile 1 day, the next day they begin kicking immediately when the ribbon is attached, indicating they used a visual cue to remind themselves (see Rovee-Collier, 1990).

Recall memory, meaning visual cues are not used, improves during the second half of the first year, a period of considerable brain development (see Chapter 27). Short-term memory grows from 2 to 10 seconds. By 9 months, babies' long-term memory for novel events extends to a day. They imitate a simple action that they witnessed yesterday, such as pressing a button to make a noise. By the time babies are crawling, they make mental maps of their surroundings, and remember where furniture should be.

Object Permanence

Piaget thought that infants did not have object permanence until at least 18 months (see **Part A**); others disagreed. Try this with a 4-month-old. Place a block on a table and put a screen in front of it within view of the baby (see **Part B**). If the screen falls forward, the baby can still see the block. If the screen falls backward, its fall is stopped by the block against which it will rest; the baby cannot see the block. Secretly remove the block so that the screen falls backward all the way. The baby will stare at this seemingly impossible event, suggesting knowledge that the block should still be present to stop the screen (Baillergeon, 1987).

Remember, Piaget's tests for object permanence required infants to physically search for objects he had hidden. Piaget did not consider the roles that neurological development, memory, or infants' impulsiveness to repeat a rewarding contingency might play in the stage 4 error.

29 Language Development

Language	Age
Crying	From birth
Cooing	2–5 mo
Babbling	5–7 mo
Single words	12 mo
Two words	18 mo
Phrases	2 yr

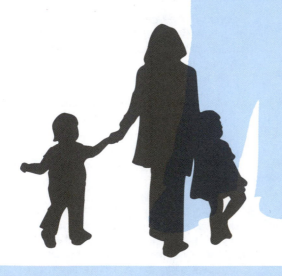

Humans are predisposed to acquire language. With no formal learning and often exposed to dramatically faulty language models, children learn words, meanings, and how to combine them in a purposeful manner.

Speech and language depend on several perceptual abilities (Owens, 1996):

1. Infants must be able to attend to speech sounds.
2. They must also be able to discriminate these sounds.
3. They must accurately remember the sequence of the speech sounds they hear.
4. They must acquire the ability to compare the sequence of speech sounds with the model they have stored in their memory.
5. They must discriminate intonational patterns.

Acquiring Language

Children acquire their language with little, if any, formal instruction and regardless of great differences in a range of social and cultural factors. This is no small achievement considering the idiosyncracies of any language. Consider some of the complexities of the English language that we, as adults, understand completely: We drive on a parkway and park on a driveway. Or think of the different sounds of letters: We eat *ghoti* quite frequently. (*gh* as in tough, *o* as in women, *ti* as in nation—put them all together and you're eating *fish*).

Key Signs of Language Development

Babies continue to learn the sounds of their language throughout the first year, and as Pinker (1994, p. 265) noted, not much of linguistic interest happens in the first 2 months. Often the coughs, cries, and hiccups during this time disturb the parents of a firstborn, but they are reflective noises indicating the baby's general physical condition (Hulit and Howard, 1997).

Too much individual variation exists to say that all children babble at 5 months, or all children utter their first words at 11 months. Babies begin to *coo* (vowel-like sounds intermingled with consonants) at the end of the second month and into the third. At about 3 or 4 months, infants begin to combine vowels and consonants to produce syllable-like sounds: *mu*, *ba*, etc. Between 5 and 7 months, these sounds appear with increasing frequency, the beginning of *babbling*. Babbling probably appears initially because of biological maturation. At 7 and 8 months, sounds like syllables appear—*da-da-da*, *ba-ba-ba* (a phenomenon occurring in all languages), a pattern that continues for the remainder of the first year (Pinker, 1994).

Late in the babbling period (usually by 9 or 10 months), children use consistent and specific sound patterns to refer to objects and events. These are called *vocables* and suggest children's discovery that meaning is associated with sound. For example, a lingering "L" sound may mean that someone is at the door.

First Words

Most children begin to speak their first words anytime from the ages of 10 to 13 months. About half of these words are for objects (food, clothing, toys). This 1-word stage may last 2 months to 1 year and has a strong relationship to words their mother uses, such as "bye-bye" or "see da da."

At 18 months children acquire words at the rate of a new word every 2 hours (a condition that lasts until about age 3 years and is frequently referred to as the *language explosion*). Vocabulary constantly expands, but estimating the extent of a child's vocabulary is difficult because youngsters know more words (their comprehension) than they say (their production). Estimates are that a 1-year-old child may use from 2 to 6 words, and a 2-year-old has a vocabulary ranging from 50 to 250 words. Children at this stage also begin to combine 2 words (Pinker, 1994).

Holophrases

You will notice a subtle change before the 2-word stage. Children begin to use 1 word to convey multiple meanings. For example, youngsters say "ball" meaning "give me the ball," "throw the ball," or "watch the ball roll." They have now gone far beyond merely labeling this round object as a ball. Often called *holophrastic speech* (use of 1 word to communicate many meanings and ideas), it is difficult to analyze. These first words, or *holophrases*, are usually nouns, adjectives, or self-inventive words and often contain multiple meanings (Dacey and Travers, 1999).

At about 18–24 months, simple 2 and 3 word sentences appear. Children primarily use nouns and verbs (not adverbs, conjunctions, or prepositions), and their sentences demonstrate grammatical structure. The initial multiple-word utterances (usually 2 or 3 words: "Timmy runs fast") are called *telegraphic speech*. Telegraphic speech contains considerably more meaning than what superficially appears in the 2 or 3 words.

Implications for Health Care Providers

If you find yourself working with children of this age, we urge you to consider the following:

- Be certain that the infant's hearing ability is normal. Children of this age should be able to distinguish speech sounds and turn toward the sound of a voice.
- Have family members help you interpret the infant's gestures and sounds.
- Use the developmental sequence presented here to help you understand the meaning of the infant's babbling and single words.
- If the infant and family are from a different culture with a different language, obtain help with both language and any cultural practices that are important for the child's recovery.

30 First Relationships

A Reciprocal interactions

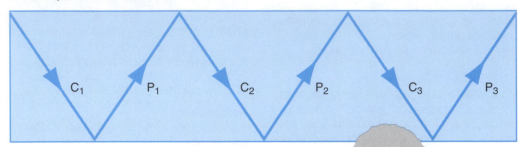

C_1 P_1 C_2 P_2 C_3 P_3

C = Child
P = Parent

B

Characteristic	Meaning
Synchrony	Refers to parents' ability to adjust their behavior to that of their children.
Symmetry	Refers to an infant's capacity for attention and style of responding, which uniquely influence any reciprocal interactions.
Contingency	Refers to the effect parents' behavior has on their infant's emotional state.
Entrainment	Refers to the rhythm established between parents and infants.
Autonomy	Refers to the time when infants realize they have a share in controlling the interactions (about 6 months of age).

Children from birth seek stimulation from their environment and instantly interpret how they are being treated. This process is called *reciprocal interactions* (see **Part A**); that is, infants react to the way they are treated and they change accordingly. As a result of the changes in babies, those around the infants (usually the parents) change.

Infants are ready to respond to social stimulation and it is not just a matter of responding passively. *Infants in their own way initiate social contacts.* Many of their actions (such as turning toward their mother or gesturing in her direction) are forms of communication. Those around infants try to attract their attention, but the babies actively select from these adult actions. In other words, infants begin to structure their own relationships according to their own unique temperaments.

What Is a Relationship?

A *relationship* implies a pattern of interactions between 2 people over an extended period of time. There are many dimensions to a relationship: the role that parents see themselves playing, their behavior, their perceptions, and their feelings for their child. What parents say or do is significant, but how their child perceives and judges that behavior is even more important. Children are excellent judges of how they are being treated.

Any relationship may be marked by apparently contradictory interactions. A mother may have a warm relationship with her child as evidenced by hugging and kissing, but she may also scold when scolding is needed for the child's protection. To understand the relationship, we must understand the interactions.

Ghosts in the Nursery

How parents were treated by *their* parents, their observation of those they consider good parents, and their reading about parenting strongly influence what they see as their parental role. Selma Fraiberg, a well-known child psychiatrist, referred to the presence of "ghosts in the nursery," which can have many consequences.

For example, some parents feel *their* parents looking over their shoulder and telling them how to bring up their child, ideas that they may well have rejected or even rebelled against. Does their child remind them of someone from the past, and do they begin to react to their child as they did to that other person? Or do they tend to imitate a friend whom they admire? Or have they been impressed by the ideas of some "expert" they have read about or seen on television? The encouraging conclusion is that in spite of these findings, when parents are aware that ghosts from the past may influence them, they are able to overcome these relics and move on to positive relations with their children.

Children's Temperament

Parental expectations as to role, however, are only one of many influences on a relationship. *Temperament* refers to a child's unique behavioral style when interacting with the environment. These differences become obvious in the first days and weeks after birth and have an immediate and decided impact on reciprocal interactions. Even mothers of identical twins will say that they can distinguish their babies by the differences in their reactions to faces, voices, various colors, and so on. Today's acceptance of the importance of inborn temperament reflects the work of two child psychiatrists, Stella Chess and Alexander Thomas (1987).

To test their ideas, Chess and Thomas conducted what came to be called the *New York Longitudinal Study* (NYLS), a study of 141 middle-class children. They found that they could draw a behavioral profile of the children by age 2 or 3 months. Certain characteristics clustered with sufficient frequency for the authors to identify 3 general types of temperament:

- **Easy children,** characterized by regularity of bodily functions, low or moderate intensity of reactions, and acceptance of, rather than withdrawal from, new situations (40% of the children).
- **Difficult children,** characterized by irregularity in bodily functions, intense reactions, and withdrawal from new stimuli (10% of the children).
- **Slow-to-warm-up children,** characterized by a low intensity of reactions and a somewhat negative mood (15% of the children).

The authors were able to classify 65% of the infants, leaving the others with a mixture of traits that defied neat categorization. Chess and Thomas also found that a *goodness of fit* existed when the demands and expectations of parents were compatible with their child's temperament, abilities, and other characteristics.

The Development of Relationships

The rhythm of the interactions between parents and their babies is the beginning of their social development. Discussing these initial interactions, the prominent pediatrician Berry Brazelton and the child psychoanalyst Bert Cramer (1990) identified several characteristics that characterize a successful relationship in the following table (see **Part B**).

Implications for Health Care Providers

As a health care provider working with infants, be alert to the quality of the relationships these babies have with their families. Given what we know today about the effect that emotions have on health, you will want to do as much as possible to provide a warm, supportive environment for infants. If you feel your options are limited in working with families, do not hesitate to turn to qualified counseling services.

31 Attachment

A The development of attachment

Age	Characteristics	Behavior
4 mo	Perceptual discrimination; visual tracking of mother.	Smiles and vocalizes more with mother than anyone else; shows distress at separation.
9 mo	Separation anxiety; stranger anxiety.	Cries when mother leaves; clings at appearance of strangers.
2–3 yr	Intensity and frequency of attachment behavior remain constant.	Notices impending departure, indicating a better understanding of surrounding world.
3–4 yr	Growing confidence; tendency to feel secure in a strange place with subordinate attachment figures (relatives).	Begins to accept mother's temporary absence; plays *with* other children.
4–10 yr	Less-intense attachment behavior, but still strong.	May hold parent's hand while walking; anything unexpected causes child to turn to parent.
Adolescence	Weakening attachment to parents; peers and other adults become important.	Becomes attached to groups and group members.
Adult	Attachment bond still discernible.	In troubled times, adults turn to trusted friends; elderly direct attention toward younger generation.

B

Adult Attachment Interview	Strange Situation Response
Secure, autonomous—Coherent; values attachment; accepts any unpleasant, earlier experiences.	Secure
Dismissing—Positive statements are unsupported or contradicted; they claim earlier unpleasant experiences have no effect.	Avoidant
Preoccupied—Seems angry, confused, passive, or fearful; some responses irrelevant.	Resistant-ambivalent
Unfocused, disorganized—Loses train of thought during discussion of loss or abuse; lapses in reasoning (speaks of dead people as alive).	Disorganized/disoriented

Attachment, the special bonding between an infant and usually the mother that develops in the first 6 months of life, is generally accepted as the foundation of social development. Infants who develop a secure attachment to their mother have the willingness and confidence to seek out future relationships. **Part A** presents the developmental stages of attachment.

The Nature of Attachment

John Bowlby and his colleagues observed a number of young children aged 15–30 months who not only were separated from their mothers, but also for weeks or months were cared for in hospitals or nurseries where they had no mother substitute. A predictable sequence of behaviors followed:

1. *Protest*, the first phase, appeared immediately and persisted for about 1 week. Loud crying, extreme restlessness, and rejection of all adult figures marked an infant's distress.
2. *Despair*, the second phase, followed next. Infants demonstrated a growing hopelessness: monotonous crying, inactivity, and steady withdrawal.
3. *Detachment*, the final phase, materialized when an infant displayed renewed interest in the surroundings, but it was a remote, distant kind of interest.

The Strange Situation

Mary Salter Ainsworth (1973) devised the "strange situation" technique to study attachment. Ainsworth brought a mother and infant to an observation room. The child was placed on the floor and allowed to play with toys. A stranger (female) then entered the room and began to talk to the mother. Observers watched to see how the infant reacted to the stranger and to what extent the child used the mother as a secure base. The mother then left the child alone in the room with the stranger; observers then noted how distressed the child became. The mother returned and the quality of the child's reaction to the mother's return was assessed. Next the infant was left completely alone, followed by the stranger's entrance, and then that of the mother. These behaviors were used to classify children as follows:

- **Securely attached infants** were secure and used the mother as a base from which to explore. These mothers were warm and consistently displayed sensitive responsiveness. During separation, the children exhibited considerable distress, ceased their explorations, and at reunion sought contact with their mothers.
- **Avoidantly attached infants** rarely cried during separation and avoided their mothers at reunion. The mothers of these babies were casual, almost indifferent, to their babies, while the babies seemed to dislike any physical contact with their mothers.

- **Ambivalently attached children** manifested anxiety before separation and were intensely distressed by the separation. These mothers were erratic with their babies, often attentive, but not sensitively responsive. On reunion the babies displayed ambivalent behavior toward their mothers; they sought contact but simultaneously seemed to resist it.
- **Disorganized/disoriented children** manifested confused behavior on being reunited with their mothers. They often looked at the mother, then looked away in a disinterested manner.

By age 7 or 8 months, when attachment behavior (as defined by Bowlby and Ainsworth) normally appears, infants are attached to both mothers and fathers and prefer either parent to a stranger.

Recent Research into Attachment

A major advance in studying attachment has been the development of the *Adult Attachment Interview* (Main, 1996). During a 1-hour interview, people are asked to furnish 5 adjectives describing their relationship to each of their own parents. Later during the interview, they are asked to give memories of specific incidents supporting these earlier answers. **Part B** illustrates the way in which the answers are categorized.

Researchers are also focusing on the relationship between early attachment and children's drawings and stories in middle childhood. When presented with instances of children who were separated from their mothers, secure 6-year-olds made up positive, constructive responses about the child in the story. But disorganized children gave frightened responses: "The mother is going to die." "The girl will kill herself."

Studies have shown an association between the way a mother recalls her childhood experiences and the present quality of the relationship with her children. Women who had been securely attached have securely attached children. The internal representations of childhood attachment seem to carry to the next generation. (See Dacey and Travers, 1999, for a further discussion of this topic.)

Implications for Health Care Providers

The contacts with mothers and their infants give nurses an opportunity to model desirable behaviors (talking to the baby, nurturing, recognizing clues to a baby's behavior). It is also an ideal time to share ideas with the mother, an exchange of views that many women find both supportive and instructive. These exchanges can be particularly valuable if the infant is preterm or ill. If the attachment process is interrupted by a hospital stay, then considerable care should be taken to explain techniques that parents can adopt to sustain the attachment process, and what to expect with regard to their own feelings and behaviors and those of their baby.

32 Emotional Development

A The development of emotions

Age	Emotions
Birth	Ability to express emotions
1–3 mo	Distress, rage, beginning of social smile
4–6 mo	Sadness, disgust, fear
7–9 mo	Joy, anger, fear, separation, and stranger anxiety

B Excitement — from birth

Distress — shortly after birth

Delight — about 3 mo

Anger, disgust, fear — about 4–6 mo

Elation — about 8 mo

Affection for adults — about 10 mo

Jealousy — about 12 mo

Affection for children — about 15 mo

Joy — from 18–24 mo

Children's emotions were long thought to be an important part of child development and in need of detailed study. Interest waned as investigators realized that neither theories nor research were sufficiently reliable to reach definite conclusions. In the last decade, however, enthusiasm about emotions and their development has returned and sparked renewed studies and speculation.

The Nature of Emotions

Daniel Goleman (1995, p. 289) defined emotion as "a feeling(s) and its distinctive thoughts, psychological and biological states, and range of propensities to act." Goleman also presented several categories of emotions, together with representative members of each family.

Anger: fury, resentment, animosity
Sadness: grief, sorrow, gloom, melancholy
Fear: nervousness, apprehension, dread, fright
Enjoyment: happiness, joy, bliss, delight
Love: acceptance, trust, devotion, adoration
Surprise: shock, astonishment, amazement, wonder
Shame: guilt, embarrassment, mortification, humiliation

Another well-known student of emotional development, Carroll Izard (1991), proposed this definition: "An emotion is experienced as a feeling that motivates, organizes, and guides perception, thought, and action." Careful examination of these definitions shows that emotion reveals 3 components:

1. First is the *feeling* that the emotion engenders. Feelings may range from pleasant to unpleasant, from enjoyment to rejection. You can induce some of the signs of an emotion—quickened breath, rapid heartbeat—but if pleasure or distress does not accompany these signs, it probably is not emotional behavior.
2. Next would be the *internal changes* associated with an emotional reaction (changes in blood pressure, heart rate, etc.).
3. Finally, there is the emotional *behavior* itself. Humans express emotional feelings by definite and specific behavioral reactions: laughing, crying, looking sad.

Signs of Emotional Development

Remember that what elicits children's emotions at different ages changes (**Part A**). Six-month-old children show amusement when tickled by their mothers, which is far different from a 16-year-old's amusement at a funny story told by a friend. Both may be labeled as "amusement," as the emotion is not the same. As children grow, the circumstances that elicit an emotion change radically.

Emotional development seems to move from the general to the specific. General positive states differentiate into such emotions as joy and interest; general negative states differentiate into fear, disgust, or anger. These primary emotions emerge during the first 6 months. Sometime after 18 months, secondary emotions that are associated with a child's growing cognitive capacity for self-awareness appear.

The differentiation of emotions is illustrated in **Part B** (Bridges, 1932). A general state of excitement is the basic emotion at birth, followed quickly by a differentiation into pleasant and unpleasant emotions. The various specific emotions continue to develop until they are recognized as responses to specific stimuli (e.g., anger to removal of a toy). Other research (Izard, 1982) suggests that interest, distress, and disgust are present at birth; anger, surprise, and sadness appear at about 3 or 4 months; fear at about 5–7 months; and shame and shyness appear at about 6–8 months.

Emotionally, infants begin to acquire a sense of trust in those around them. This ability reaches a peak between ages 4 and 6 months (Greenspan, 1995). During these months, children who experience upsetting conditions (rough handling, chaotic feeding patterns, overstimulation) learn that they cannot depend on their environment. Mistrust begins to develop.

At about 6 months, children start to react to the facial expressions of those around them, to read body language, and to recognize any tensions in their surroundings. Gradually their nonverbal communication skills sharpen and they begin to understand the basics of human interactions from about 12 to 18 months (Greenspan, 1995).

The Smile

A baby's smile is one of the first signs of emotion. Most parents immediately interpret a smile as a sign of happiness. However, early smiles do not have the social significance of the smile that emerges at about 6 weeks. These early smiles are usually designated as "false" smiles because they lack the emotional warmth of the true smile. By the baby's third week, the human female voice elicits a brief, real smile. By the sixth week the true social smile appears, especially in response to the human face.

Implications For Health Care Providers

In your interactions with your clients, you will encounter a wide range of emotions, from fear and anxiety to outright anger. Recognizing the components of emotion–feelings, internal changes, and behavior–will guide your reactions to a person's behavior. Your analysis of the emotion(s) expressed will help you decide whether support, encouragement, or firmness is needed. By maintaining an open and honest relationship with clients, you will be able to help them, not only with their physical problems, but any emotional difficulties as well.

PART III: QUESTIONS

Directions: For each of the following questions, choose the **one best** answer.

1. At what point after birth do typical infants double their birth weight?

(A) 3 months

(B) 6 months

(C) 9 months

(D) 12 months

2. You notice that a new mother feeds her baby boy by propping a bottle on a pillow next to him. Why do you want to discourage this practice?

(A) The baby will have difficulty regulating the flow of formula.

(B) The baby is not learning how to organize his behavior.

(C) Mother and baby are not learning to read each other's signals.

(D) All of the above are correct.

3. You observe a baby lying on her abdomen, raising her head, shoulders, and upper abdomen while supporting herself with her forearms. About how old is this baby?

(A) 6 weeks

(B) 8 weeks

(C) 3 months

(D) 6 months

4. A new mother who is breast-feeding her baby asks you if her baby can see her. What is your answer?

(A) "No. Babies can't see clearly until they're about 6 weeks old."

(B) "Yes. Babies have 20/20 vision at birth."

(C) "No. Visual acuity is about 20/100 at birth."

(D) "Yes. Objects that are within close range, especially your face, are perfectly clear."

5. Apgar scores are recorded at 1 and 5 minutes after birth. What do they measure?

(A) Heart rate, respiratory effort, muscle tone, reflex irritability, and skin color

(B) First and second periods of reactivity

(C) Behavioral states: sleeping, waking, and crying

(D) Gestational maturity, such as flexion of extremities, quality of skin, and development of eyes, ears, and genitals

6. Which of the following is an example of contingency seeking in newborns?

(A) Infants learn to adjust their rate of sucking using the mother's voice as a reward.

(B) Infants prefer complex patterns of black and white.

(C) Newborns discriminate their mother's voice from that of other women.

(D) Infants turn their head to search for a sound.

7. The final area of the brain to develop is the

(A) occipital lobe.

(B) association area.

(C) sensory area.

(D) auditory area.

8. Nervous system development commences in a process called

(A) neural induction.

(B) tubular processes.

(C) neural migration.

(D) neuronal balance.

9. Human infants exhibit reflexes because

(A) their nervous systems are not fully mature.

(B) some infant reflexes are building blocks for voluntary motor behavior.

(C) some reflexes are designed to protect them from potential harm.

(D) of all of the above.

10. To elicit the Babinski reflex, you stroke the sole of a baby's foot, beginning at the heel and moving toward the toes. The toes flex, as if they are going to grab your finger. Is this normal?

(A) No. If the baby is less than 1 year old, the toes should fan out and extend.

(B) Yes. If the baby is over 1 year old, the toes will flex.

(C) Both A and B are true.

(D) Neither A nor B is true.

11. According to Piaget, what are the 4 accomplishments of the sensorimotor period?

(A) Rolling over, sitting up, crawling, and walking

(B) Time, spatial relationships, cause and effect, and object permanence

(C) Visual acuity, binocular vision, depth perception, and spatial relationships

(D) Primary circular reactions, secondary circular reactions, coordination of secondary circular reactions, and tertiary circular reactions

12. You are watching a baby who is sitting up in her mother's lap. The baby is playing with a box of animal crackers, shaking it, hitting it on the arm of the chair, and patting the lid with her hand. What age range and what substage of Piaget's sensorimotor period is this baby in?

(A) Age 1–4 months, primary circular reactions

(B) Age 4–8 months, secondary circular reactions

(C) Age 8–12 months, coordination of secondary circular reactions

(D) Age 18–24 months, beginning of representational thought

13. A significant feature of early language development is its

(A) unique pattern.

(B) receptivity.

(C) evocative nature.

(D) pitch.

14. Most children begin to speak their first words at about

(A) 6 months.

(B) 12 months.

(C) 18 months.

(D) 24 months.

15. Which of the following statements is incorrect?

(A) Children instantly tune into their environment.

(B) Children give clues to their personalities.

(C) Children, from birth, engage in reciprocal interactions.

(D) All children are temperamentally similar at birth.

16. *Role* refers to _____ about behavior.

(A) observations

(B) insights

(C) expectations

(D) comments

17. That special bonding between an infant and usually the mother is called

(A) detachment.

(B) attachment.

(C) relating.

(D) symmetry.

18. The person most associated with the attachment movement is

(A) Sigmund Freud.

(B) B. F. Skinner.

(C) Jean Piaget.

(D) John Bowlby.

19. The components of an emotion are feelings, internal changes, and

(A) behavior.

(B) continuity.

(C) congruence.

(D) assimilation.

20. The true social smile appears at

(A) 4 weeks.

(B) 6 weeks.

(C) 8 weeks.

(D) 10 weeks.

PART III: ANSWERS AND EXPLANATIONS

1. The answer is B.

The average American newborn weighs 3.27 kg. Infants gain 680 g a month until about age 5–6 months, by which time their birth weight has doubled. Birth weight triples by the end of the first year, to about 10 kg.

2. The answer is D.

Feeding, especially breast-feeding, is a learned behavior that contributes to self-regulation in infants and sensitive responding in mothers. Mothers and infants learn to coordinate supply and demand of milk, especially during the first few weeks of life. This give-and-take requires that mothers learn to read infants' signals of hunger, fatigue, distress, and satisfaction. As infants learn to regulate the flow of milk, they also learn to organize their own behavior. Feeding, especially at the breast, helps them to calm down and focus. An attentive infant in the arms of a responsive mother is ready to interact with her, to focus his or her eyes on her face and listen to her voice.

3. The answer is C.

Head control is a good indicator of brain maturation. Newborns cannot lift their heads until they are 6 weeks old, and then do so briefly. By 3–4 months, they raise their head, shoulders, and upper abdomen while supporting themselves on their forearms. When newborns are pulled to sit, their head falls back. Head lag decreases and infants have steady head control by 5–6 months, when they can sit with support.

4. The answer is D.

At birth, visual acuity is about 20/100 and steadily improves. Newborns can see and fixate on objects within 20 cm of the center of their bodies. That means that objects within close range, like the mother's face, are perfectly clear. A preference for patterns is evident within hours after birth. Patterns that are somewhat complex and that have moving parts, especially the human face, are of greatest interest.

5. The answer is A.

Apgar scores are used as a rough assessment of immediate adjustment to extrauterine life. Heart rate, respirations, muscle tone, reflexes, and skin color are assessed at 1 and 5 minutes after birth, with each given a score of 0, 1, or 2. Total scores less than 3 indicate severe distress. Scores of 4–6 signify moderate difficulty, and scores of 7–10 indicate no difficulty adapting to extrauterine life. Apgar scores are affected by

prematurity and maternal medication, and are not indicative of the presence or absence of neurological or physical abnormalities.

6. The answer is A.

Newborn behavior has 4 characteristics. Inborn physiological mechanisms, such as reflexes, enhance survival. Newborns organize their behavior in response to stimuli (e.g., turning their head in response to a sound). They respond selectively to certain stimuli (e.g., patterns of light and dark). Newborns demonstrate contingency-seeking behavior; that is, they look for predictability in the environment, for events that go together. In a classic experiment, DeCasper demonstrated that infants learn to adjust their rate of sucking using the mother's voice as a reward. That is, infants learned that hearing their mother's voice was contingent on how fast they sucked on a pacifier.

7. The answer is B.

The complex cognitive activities that slowly appear throughout development are rooted in the association area and testify to the interaction between body and mind.

8. The answer is A.

Once neural induction begins, the process is swift and steady. Any interference with the process (disease, chemicals) can produce serious damage.

9. The answer is D.

The CNS is not fully developed at birth, and continues to grow, reorganize, and mature. The specialized regions that give rise to reflexes are found in the more primitive areas of the CNS, such as the spinal cord, brain stem, and cerebellum. Some adaptive infant reflexes are building blocks for voluntary motor behaviors that develop with experience and with maturity of the cortical regions of the brain. Thus, reflexes can also provide a window into neurological development because they should change as the nervous system matures. Finally, some reflexes—like blinking—are permanent throughout life, designed to protect humans from potential harm.

10. The answer is C.

The Babinski reflex is an example of how reflexes change as the nervous system matures. In infants, the toes fan out and extend, and there is dorsiflexion of the big toe. By age 1 year, the reflexive fanning out disappears, and is replaced by the mature response found in children and adults. The toes flex when the sole of the foot is stroked.

11. The answer is B.

By "sensorimotor," Piaget meant that mental life begins with infants' ability to interact with the physical environment using their bodies. Physical actions are accompanied by a growing awareness by infants of how their behavior affects the environment. The 4 accomplishments of this period are (1) spatial relationships—in and out, up and down, near and far; (2) time—before and after; (3) causality—cause and effect, one event inevitably leads to another; and (4) object permanence—objects exist when out of sight.

12. The answer is B.

During the substage of secondary circular reactions, about age 4–8 months, infants use their bodies to act on the physical environment (secondary), repeating actions (circular) because they produce a desired effect. Infants realize they can make things happen. Examples include shaking a rattle, hitting a hanging toy to make it swing, and patting and squeezing toys.

13. The answer is B.

The quality of the language surrounding children affects many aspects of development. Talking *to* a child, not *at* a child, provides a rich, stimulating environment.

14. The answer is B.

Although first words usually are spoken at about 1 year, parents should not be disturbed if language is delayed. The best advice is to watch this phase of development carefully and seek advice if any delay is worrisome.

15. The answer is D.

Research has shown that children's personalities are unique from birth. This conclusion offers clues for parents to use in establishing positive interactions with their children.

16. The answer is C.

People associate certain characteristics with individuals, tasks, occupations, etc. They then formulate expectations about these characteristics.

17. The answer is B.

Most developmental psychologists believe that attachment is the basis for social development. Once again, the importance of the initial interactions between parent and child is emphasized.

18. The answer is D.

Bowlby's work on children's first relationships made psychologists aware of the significance of the initial interactions for future social development.

19. The answer is A.

We judge emotional behavior by what we see. Emotions are characterized by specific types of behavior—joy, sadness, etc.

20. The answer is B.

Many developmental features come together at about 6 weeks for babies to display a true social smile. In addition, psychosocial and cognitive factors interact to enable a baby to display the smile.

PART IV
Early Childhood

33 Growth and Motor Development

A Height and weight measurements: 50th percentiles

Age (yr)	Boys		Girls	
	Height (cm)	Weight (kg)	Height (cm)	Weight (kg)
$2\frac{1}{2}$	90.4	13.53	90	13.03
3	94.9	14.62	94.1	14.1
$3\frac{1}{2}$	99.1	15.68	97.9	15.07
4	102.9	16.69	101.6	15.96
$4\frac{1}{2}$	106.6	17.69	105	16.81
5	109.9	18.67	108.4	17.66
6	116.1	20.69	114.6	19.52

B Motor development

Age	Gross Motor	Fine Motor	General Physical
3	Rides tricycle Jumps, climbs, kicks Stands on 1 foot for a few seconds Goes up stairs alternating feet, down using 2 feet	Builds tower of 9 cubes Adept at placing pellet into a narrow-necked bottle In drawing, copies strokes Draws a face using a circle Uses fork	Average weight 14.6 kg (32 lb) Average height 95 cm (37.2 inches) May have achieved nighttime control of bowel and bladder Vision is 20/30
4	Skips, hops on 1 foot Catches a ball with 2 hands Walks down stairs alternating feet	Uses kiddie scissors Can lace shoes, cannot tie In drawing, copies square Adds 3 parts to stick figure	Average weight 16.7 kg (37 lb) Average height 103 cm (40.5 inches) Length at birth is doubled Vision is 20/20
5	Skips, hops alternating feet Jumps rope Ice skates with balance Throws, catches ball well	Uses scissors, pencil well Ties shoelaces, buttons Draws stick figure Prints some letters/numbers	Average weight 18.7 kg (41 lb) Average height 110 cm (43 inches) Handedness is established May start to lose baby teeth
6	Very active physically Runs up and down stairs May ride bicycle Throws ball overhand	Cuts, folds, pastes Uses knife to spread jam Knows right from left Likes to draw, color	Weight 16–23 kg (35–58 lb) Height 106–123 cm (42–48 inches) Permanent teeth erupting, can brush them

The rate of growth slows during the preschool years. Children gain about 2.3 kg (5 lb) each year, and grow taller by 6.0–7.5 cm (2–3 inches) per year. (see **Parts A** and **B**). There are few physical differences between boys and girls during this time, however, there is increasing variability among individual children.

While most of the increase in height occurs in the legs, the chubby pot-bellied body of the toddler gives way to a more slender and posturally erect profile. Preschoolers are better coordinated than their younger selves. By age 3, children are walking, running, jumping, and climbing well. Their sense of balance improves markedly. A 3-year-old can stand on 1 foot for a few seconds; by age 4, the same child is hopping around on 1 foot. At 3 years, most children are riding a tricycle; by 6 years, many have mastered riding a 2-wheel bike. At 3 years, children can go upstairs using alternating feet, but still descend placing both feet on each step. By age 4, they descend using alternating feet, holding the railing. At age 6, they are running up and down stairs easily (see **Part B**).

Muscles and bones are not yet fully developed, however. While most preschoolers appear sturdy, able, and motivated, they are not physically ready for athletic activities that require endurance and coordination for sustained periods of time. This age group is also reckless due to lack of judgment and impulsiveness. Injuries are the leading cause of death between ages 1 and 4.

Fine-motor skills also improve markedly as preschoolers use their hands as tools (see **Part B**). They enjoy projects that involve finger painting, playing with Play-Doh, pasting, and coloring. They build with blocks, put together large-piece puzzles, and zoom little cars around toy villages. They button and zip, although tying shoelaces takes much practice.

Visuomotor Development: Hand-eye Coordination and Drawing

Vision is 20/20 by age 4. Children also become more efficient and proficient in how they move their eyes to scan a page, an ability essential for reading readiness. At age 3, when asked to find an object or the page of a book, children initially scan haphazardly, looking here and there. Systematic scanning side to side and up and down develops between ages 3 and 6.

The combination of perceptual development and fine-motor development produces the ability to hold a pencil or crayon for the purposes of drawing, tracing, and copying pictures, letters, and numbers. Three-year-old children can copy a picture of a circle, and will draw crude facial features in it, but left to themselves, they scribble. By age 4, they copy a square, and are more adept at tracing shapes, such as a cross or diamond. While not adept at drawing human stick figures, they can add a few parts, like arms and legs, to one partially drawn for them. At age 5, they add more detail to stick figures, like fingers, hair, and earrings. In kindergarten, children can copy most basic shapes, and trace and print numbers and letters.

Brain Development

Handedness, improvement in fine- and gross-motor skills, and advances in cognitive development (see Chapter 32) are related to maturational changes in the brain and spinal cord. Neural development is of 2 kinds: growth and organization. The number of synapses and amount of myelin increase in several major areas of the brain simultaneously between ages 2 and 5, with a spurt occurring between 5 and 7 years. At age 3, the brain is 50% of its adult weight; by age 6, it has reached 90%. How the different areas communicate with one another and coordinate activity accounts for behavioral changes.

Take riding a bike. Improvement in balance is attributed not just to growth of the cerebellum (more synapses), but also to its ability to organize information about where the body is in space and how it is moving based on signals from muscles, joints, the semicircular canals of the inner ear, and perceptual systems (vision, hearing, sensation). The ability to regain balance rests in the thalamus, which in coordination with the neocortex regulates arousal by calling attention to relevant information, such as changes in road surface. This means a 6-year-old can learn to ride a 2-wheel bike; a 3-year-old cannot.

The neocortex is the last part of the human brain to evolve but accounts for 75% of its neurons. It is responsible for higher-level functions, such as thought and emotion. The neocortex is divided into the right and left hemispheres. Handedness, which is established by age 6, is generally believed to be a function of lateralization; that is, it becomes localized in either the right or the left hemisphere of the brain (Springer and Deutsch, 1997).

The frontal lobes are associated with changes in cognitive-emotional development (Case, 1992) including the ability to regulate attention, develop short-term memory strategies, and regulate behavior and feelings. Improvements in these abilities correspond to changes in brain wave patterns on an electroencephalograph (EEG).

Developmental Delay

Developmental delay refers to a significant lag in 1 or more of 4 areas: gross-motor coordination, fine-motor and visuomotor coordination, language, and social behaviors (Capute and Accardo, 1996). Delays in fine-motor and visuomotor skills may not be apparent until the preschool years, and can complicate developmental progress in other areas. Children who have difficulty building with blocks or cutting and pasting have trouble playing with peers, which can lead to frustration and inappropriate behaviors. Developmental screening is routinely done as part of well-child visits during the preschool years.

34 Cognitive Development—Part A

A

Characteristics	Examples
Centration	Focus on one aspect of something at a time, e.g., how much juice in a glass depends on either width or height but not both.
Perceptually bound	Deal with appearances, cannot work out a problem in their minds; not impressed by magic tricks because they do not appreciate the trick.
Cause by association	If two events happen close together, one is assumed to have caused the other.
Lack of conservation: mass	Thinks a ball of clay gets bigger when it is rolled into a snake.
Lack of conservation: number	Given 2 rows of 10 M&Ms each, will say the row that is more spread out contains more.
Lack of conservation: quantity	Says the glass with the most juice is the taller one, even if the child just saw it poured from a shorter but wider glass.
Classification	Classify objects based on only 1 aspect of them, e.g., color, size.

B

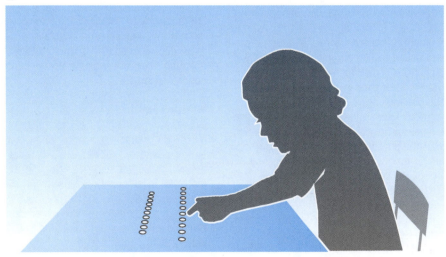

Preoperational Period

Piaget referred to the period from ages 2½ to about 6 as "preoperational" or "prelogical" because it precedes the period of concrete operations that is associated with the school-age years, roughly ages 7–11. Preschoolers think about things in ways that infants and toddlers do not. They represent ideas in their minds. They recognize that physical events have explanations, although their explanations may not make sense. Preschool-aged children try to figure things out. There are limitations in their ability to reason logically. Preoperational thinking is referred to as "magical," meaning children's ideas about how the world works can be quite fanciful and are not grounded in the principles of physics (**Part A**). A young child truly believes he or she can disappear down the bathtub drain preoperational thinking.

Centration

The children focus on only 1 aspect of something at a time—often the most obvious aspect—and fail to consider how several aspects might interact to produce the event. When pouring juice between a tall skinny glass and a short wide glass, they focus on only the height of the tall skinny glass in concluding that it is "bigger" and so contains more juice. They cannot account for height and width simultaneously.

Appearance-reality Problem

Preschool children are perceptually bound; that is, they deal with what appears to be true. "What you see is what you get." Santa can be in the mall and on the sidewalk at the same time because they saw him in both places. The sun truly goes down into the ground at night.

Cause by Association

Causality is explained in a circular fashion, without distinguishing between cause and effect. If 2 events appear to happen at the same time, one is believed to have caused the other, although children cannot explain how. Children believe they catch cold from being outside in winter. Cause by association also explains why some adults think AIDS can be transmitted by shaking hands. It can just happen.

Difficulty with Conservation

Conservation refers to the ability to understand that something remains the same even if its appearance is altered and nothing was seen to be taken away or added. Because preschool children are swayed by appearances, focus on 1 aspect of something at a time, and have difficulty working out events in their minds, they have difficulty with conservation tasks.

Conservation of number is the ability to recognize that a set of items remains the same in number despite being rearranged. Preschoolers are not so sure. For example, in an experiment to test for perceptually bound thinking and lack of conservation of number, present a child with 2 rows of M&Ms with 10 in each row. In 1 row, bunch the M&Ms closely together (see **Part B**). In the second row, spread them apart so that when side by side the second row extends beyond the first. Ask the child which row has more M&Ms. Why? The child will focus on the length of a row, deciding that the longer of 2 rows has "more." If small numbers of items—3 or 4 items—are used, the child demonstrates conservation skills.

Conservation of quantity is recognizing that liquids take the form of their containers; a cup of water is a cup of water regardless if it is in a tall or short glass. Again, preschoolers will focus on the height of the tall glass in concluding it contains "more," even if children pour the water back and forth between the 2 glasses themselves. They cannot mentally reverse this action and conceptualize that the quantity of water stays the same. They also cannot compensate height for width.

Conservation of mass and/or length is the ability to understand that the appearance of solid objects can be altered yet their mass and/or length remains the same. Preschoolers think that a ball of Play-Doh gets bigger when it is rolled into a snake. They are sure that a ball of string pulled out to its full length grows longer.

Classification

If a preschooler were asked to help sort belongings from a closet, they might put a shoe and shirt together because they are both red, then add a blue belt because it has a buckle like the shoe. Classification is initially based on saliency, that is, what is obvious, what appeals at the time. By kindergarten, children begin to understand class inclusion. For example, shoes, sneakers, and boots are footwear; a shirt does not belong.

35 Cognitive Development—Part B

A

Characteristics	Examples
Centration	Focus on one aspect of something at a time, e.g., how much juice in a glass depends on either width or height but not both.
Perceptually bound	Deal with appearances, cannot work out a problem in their minds; not impressed by magic tricks because they do not appreciate the trick.
Cause by association	If two events happen close together, one is assumed to have caused the other.
Lack of conservation: mass	Thinks a ball of clay gets bigger when it is rolled into a snake.
Lack of conservation: number	Given 2 rows of 10 M&Ms each, will say the row that is more spread out contains more.
Lack of conservation: quantity	Says the glass with the most juice is the taller one, even if the child just saw it poured from a shorter but wider glass.
Classification	Classify objects based on only 1 aspect of them, e.g., color, size.

B

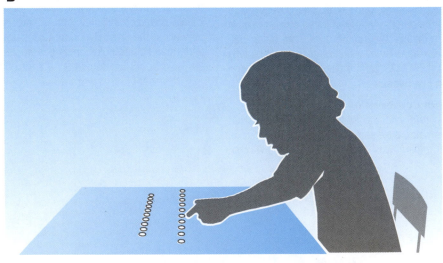

Alternatives to Piaget

Piaget's reliance on a verbal explanation of events is a major weakness in his theory. As noted in the chapter on infant cognition, the nature of the task used to investigate how children think can influence the results. For example, compare 2 seriation tasks: ordering sticks according to length and stacking measuring cups inside of one another. For the sticks, children use trial and error, and cannot focus on 2 things at once—length of stick and its relationship to what is before and after it. They can "complete" the task incorrectly. For the cups, there is only 1 correct solution. The task tells them when they are wrong, and encourages children to "reverse" the results of incorrect trials, if not in their minds then with their hands. They successfully seriate the cups because the task provides "error information," that is, the big one cannot fit into the little one. Seriating sticks does not provide that kind of feedback.

During the preschool years, there are improvements in both how much children remember and how they remember it. Capacity improves due to maturation of the neocortex and the explosion in language skills. Words help children to construct a useful network of associations about things, which is called *encoding*. They store this network in long-term memory, which appears to be unlimited over their lifetimes. Short-term memory lengthens to 30 seconds but is limited to 3–5 pieces of information. The short-term capacity of an older child or adult is 7–9.

Memory strategies improve markedly, but are not as efficient as in older children. Ask a young child to remember a phone number: 555-1234. Seven digits exceeds their short-term capacity, and they have trouble chunking the number into 2 pieces of information—555 and 1234—which older children can do. So they might rehearse it out loud. But a clue—it starts with 555—will jog their memory. However, if the phone number is set to a familiar tune, children will remember it better because songs and music are stored whole in a different area of the brain.

Adults are often amazed by young children's memory. Keep in mind they remember what they pay attention to and they pay attention to what is salient. Their network of associations can be fanciful. A 4-year-old girl will remember what you wore to a family wedding, but may forget whose wedding it was.

Implications for Health Care Providers

A preoperational explanation of illness is based on association of events. The illness is described as its symptoms. A cold is when the nose runs. An external cause may be identified, but children cannot explain how cause leads to effect. A cold is from being outside in the winter (Bibace and Walsh, 1981). Illness can "just happen," out of the child's control. Use associations to manage the treatment regimen: Take medicine at bedtime. Take their fears seriously.

Early Childhood Education

Biopsychosocial interactions

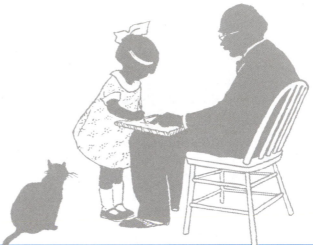

Bio	Psycho	Social
Genetics	Cognitive development	Attachment
Fertilization	Information processing	Relationships
Pregnancy	Problem solving	Reciprocal interactions
Birth	Perceptual development	School
Physical development	Language development	Peers
Motor development	Moral development	Television
Puberty	Self-efficacy	Stress
Menstruation	Personality	Marriage
Disease	Body image	Family

The growing demand for early education (preschool and kindergarten programs) is testimony to the critical importance of education during the early years. The *National Association for the Education of Young Children* (NAEYC) has defined an early childhood education program as any group program in a center, school, or other facility that serves children from birth through age 8 (Bredekamp and Copple, 1997).

Today's programs are not exclusively social or cognitive; typically elements of both occur in all programs (Dacey and Travers, 1999). Developmentally appropriate practices are based on data from 3 sources: *child development and learning*, the *characteristics of individual children*, and the *contexts* in which children develop.

The Importance of Biopsychosocial Interactions

In today's early childhood education programs, children are encouraged to learn through interacting with their environments and to be active participants in constructing knowledge. To help children achieve this goal, developmental psychologists have adopted a *biopsychosocial model* (see **Table**).

Several important biological, psychological, and social characteristics affect growth during early childhood. More importantly, however, the *interactions* that occur among the 3 categories are particularly crucial. To give a simple example, genetic damage (biological) may negatively affect cognitive development (psychological) and lead to poor peer relationships (social).

Among those who have contributed to the knowledge of developmentally appropriate practices for early childhood programs are Montessori, Piaget, and Vygotsky.

Montessori and the Absorbent Mind

Maria Montessori (1967) was a strong proponent of early childhood programs. She believed that developing children pass through different physical and mental growth phases that alternate with periods of transition. These phases, called *sensitive periods*, signify when children are especially ready for certain types of learning.

Montessori described 3 major periods of development: the absorbent mind phase, the uniform growth phase, and the adolescent phase. The *absorbent mind phase*, extending from birth to age 6, indicates a child's tremendous ability to absorb, rapidly and effortlessly, experiences from the environment.

From about 3 to 6 years, children mainly learn by doing. As they play with their Lego sets, for example, they manipulate the individual parts and begin to understand how things go together and how one series of actions becomes the basis for another.

Montessori, working with the poor children of Rome, believed that a *prepared environment* was necessary

because most children do not live in ideal surroundings. Children love order and receive satisfaction and develop feelings of security from perceiving and interacting with an ordered environment.

Piaget and Preschool Programs

Perhaps Piaget's main contribution to the development of early childhood programs was his recognition that children are quite different from adults in several important ways, especially their views of reality and their use of language. Since a child's world is qualitatively different from an adult's, the notion of *developmentally appropriate practices* takes on special meaning. Touching, feeling, and tasting are critical to cognitive development as children construct their own worlds (which is the meaning of *constructivism*).

Children who delight in swinging, in building castles in the sand, or in using the parallel bars are learning more than the muscular coordination needed. They are also learning about the needed momentum to swing higher, about the texture of sand, or about the smoothness of the bar's metal. In a piagetian-oriented preschool program, play and games are devised to promote physical, cognitive, and social development.

Vygotsky and Early Childhood Education

For Vygotsky (see Chapter 4), the basic psychological mechanism in development is social interaction, which encourages development through the guidance of skillful adults. A child's zone of proximal development (see Chapter 4) should constantly guide an instructor's work. The importance of *scaffolding* in early childhood programs reflects Vygotsky's concerns with the nature of children's environments.

Implications for Health Care Providers

The following guidelines offer a blueprint for working with early childhood youngsters (Bredekamp and Copple, 1997):

- *Create a caring community of learners*. Developmentally appropriate practices support the development of relationships among children, adults, and families.
- Try to provide the means for an interactive environment, one that encourages children to construct their own understanding of their world.
- Remember also that children's development requires multiple, ongoing assessments that are directed at specific goals and reflect children's individual differences.
- Finally, if an early education program is to be successful, then detailed knowledge of children is vital. Parents are obviously a vital source of data, and a family-centered orientation with parents and professionals working together to achieve shared goals offers the most promising means of ensuring children's maximum growth.

37 Language Development

A The pattern of vocabulary development

Age (yr)	No. of Words
2	250+
$2\frac{1}{2}$	500+
3	1,000
$3\frac{1}{2}$	1,250
4	1,600
$4\frac{1}{2}$	1,900
5	2,000
$5\frac{1}{2}$	2,500
6	3,000

B

Rules	Meaning
Phonology	How to put sounds together to form words.
Syntax	How to put words together to form sentences.
Semantics	How to interpret the meaning of words.
Pragmatics	How to take part in a conversation.

From about ages 2 to 6 years, language figuratively "explodes." The steady progression in vocabulary development is evident in **Part A**. Children of 5 years seem to know about 2,000 words, but that is not the limit of their vocabulary. These same children *understand* many more words than they use. From the first year, children show an ability for *receptive language* (i.e., they receive and understand the words). In early childhood, they produce language themselves, *expressive language*.

Psychologists, using fairly simple strategies, estimate that today's typical high school graduate knows 45,000 words, more than 3 times Shakespeare's vocabulary. Based on these same techniques, a 6-year-old child probably *knows* as many as 10,000–15,000 words.

The Process of Language Acquisition

By the time they are ready to enter kindergarten, most children have a vocabulary of about 10,000 words. They use questions, negative statements, and dependent clauses, and have learned to use language in a variety of social situations.

Language as Rule Learning

Children deduce the rules they must follow to use words and put words together to make sentences. While this is going on, they are also learning the correct way to combine words, the rules or grammar of their language. The rules describe the relationships between sounds, between words, between words and meaning, and between words and the purpose of communication (Owens, 1996). These rules (see **Part B**) make language a powerful human tool.

The number of sentences that can be generated from English, with its thousands of nouns, verbs, adjectives, adverbs, prepositions, and conjunctions, staggers the imagination.

The Pattern of Language Development

During early childhood, children develop their language as follows:

- *2 years old.* Children's vocabularies expand rapidly, and simple 2- and 3-word sentences begin to appear: Me go, Timmy eat. These are referred to as *telegraphic speech*, and may contain multiple meanings. Children primarily use nouns and verbs, and their sentences show grammatical structure. They use the same organizational principles as adults.
- *3 years old.* Children are reaching the end of the language explosion and although their sentences may sound ungrammatical, they are actually obeying the rules with astonishing regularity. They use correct word order and inflections where required. As Pinker (1994) noted, 3-year-olds are grammatical geniuses: They master most constructions, they consistently obey language rules, and even their mistakes occur because they follow the rules *too* strictly (Janey runned to the door).
- *4 years old.* Children have acquired the complicated structure of their native tongue, are using more complex sentences (4 or 5 words), and ask ceaseless questions. (How many times have you been asked, "Why?" by a child of this age?)
- *5–6 years old.* As children come to the end of early childhood, they speak and understand sentences that they have never previously used or heard. They have become sophisticated language users, which is not to say that their language is flawless.

Language Irregularities

Certain irregularities are to be expected during these years. For example, *overextensions* mark children's beginning words. Assume that a child has learned the name of the house pet, "doggy." Think what that label means: an animal with a head, tail, body, and 4 legs. Now consider what other animals "fit" this label: cats, horses, donkeys, and cows. Consequently, children may briefly apply "doggy" to all 4-legged creatures, but they quickly eliminate overextensions.

Overregularities are a similar fleeting phenomenon. As youngsters begin to use 2- and 3-word sentences, they struggle to convey more precise meanings by mastering the grammatical rules of their language. For example, for many English verbs, the suffix *ed* is added to indicate past tense: "I want to play ball." "I wanted to play ball." But for other verbs the form is changed much more radically: "Did Daddy *come* home?" "Daddy *came* home." Most children, even after they have mastered the correct form of such verbs as come, see, and run, still add *ed* to the original form. That is, youngsters who know that the past tense of *come* is *came* will still say, "Daddy *comed* home."

Implications for Health Care Providers

In working with children of this age, you should be alert to the possibility of hearing problems. Children use their hearing to learn the language and speech skills necessary for social interaction and academic success. Hearing-impaired children possess the same potential for acquiring language as other children, but they lack linguistic input, the raw material of language.

Estimates are that about 8% of Americans, or over 17 million children and adults, experience some form of hearing difficulty. Within this group, approximately 100,000 are preschool youngsters.

38 Role of the Family

A

Values:
How well will my child do?
Examples: achievement, status, maturity

Economics:
Will my child support himself/herself and a family?
Examples: learn a trade, farm, go to school

Survival:
Will my child grow up?
Threats: disease, violence, environmental hazards

B Parenting styles

	Warm, Nurturing	Responsive?	Maturity Demands	Discipline	Child Self-control	Child: Social
Authoritarian	Maybe	No	High, clearly stated	Power assertive	External locus, aggressive	Polite, not prosocial
Authoritative	Yes	Yes	High, clearly negotiated	Inductive reasoning	Internal locus, self-control	Competent, prosocial
Permissive/ neglectful	No	No	None, unclear	None	Poor, very aggressive	Poor or no social skills
Permissive/ indulgent	Maybe	Maybe	Low, inconsistent	Avoids	Low, aggressive at home	Not prosocial, responsible

The family is the primary social group in which children learn to exercise self-control, develop empathy, and behave appropriately.

Parenting Behaviors

Authoritarian parents aim to control their children's behavior by enforcing absolute standards for behavior. They value unquestioned respect for and compliance with authority, and discourage verbal give-and-take with their children. Authoritarian parents resolve conflicts through power assertion; that is, they lay down the law "or else." They may be warm, but not responsive. Their children lack spontaneity, are overly polite, and develop an external locus of control, meaning they perceive powerful others to be responsible for events. Thus, personal initiative and prosocial behaviors are not valued or exhibited. Boys in particular have lower self-esteem. They experience power assertion as punishment, and are aggressive outside of the home but not necessarily within the family.

Authoritative parents also make high demands on their children but they are more responsive. They expect mature behavior from their children and actively guide them toward that end. Standards are clear and enforced through contingencies; that is, children are held responsible for the foreseeable consequences of their decisions. This requires some verbal give-and-take, during which parents use inductive reasoning to help children think through their actions. Discipline meted out in this way is not experienced as punitive. Children grow up to be socially competent, friendly, with good self-esteem. Their internal locus of control allows them to believe they are responsible for events, and so they take initiative and are achievement oriented. They are more prosocial than other children, and less aggressive.

Permissive parents are either indulgent or neglectful. They have few rules, which are unclear and not consistently enforced, and make few demands on their children regarding mature behavior. Neglectful parents avoid interactions with their children, whereas indulgent parents avoid circumstances in which they might have to discipline them. Indulgent parents may be warm and responsive but resolve conflicts by letting the children do as they want. These children are immature, have low self-control and a diminished sense of responsibility, and cannot rely on their own judgment. Children who have been indulged exhibit aggressive behavior at home but not in the community. Children who have been neglected are aggressive in both places, have poor self-control, and have difficulty functioning in society.

While parenting style is usually consistent within a family over time, individual parents occasionally deviate from their own style. Circumstances outside of the family also contribute to parenting style. In hostile environments that threaten children's well-being, such as inner cities or civil unrest, an authoritarian style of parenting can be more adaptive.

Siblings

As a child's first peers, siblings are important socializing agents (Dunn, 1992). Young children develop affection for the new baby, provide comfort, and protect. Infants become attached to older siblings as they do to parents.

The interactions between siblings are different from that of children and parents. Whereas conversations between parents and children focus on caregiving and discipline, siblings talk about feelings and their own wants in a playful way. When conflict arises, they lobby for their own point of view. Taking another's viewpoint into consideration while resolving conflict to their mutual benefit is a key task in moral and social development.

Older siblings provide more effective scaffolding for younger siblings than do peers. When asked to help a younger sibling with a hands-on project, older siblings provide more explanations and encouragement, and let the younger child have more control. The younger child asks more questions of and demands more control from an older sibling than a peer. Older siblings feel a sense of pride when their younger siblings succeed under their tutelage.

Warm parenting and secure parent-child attachments foster positive sibling interactions, whereas cold and intrusive parenting fosters sibling antagonism. Parents who are hostile and use power assertive discipline promote aggression between their offspring.

Determinants of Parenting

Responsive parenting is like money in the bank. It pays dividends for years to come. Three factors determine how people parent their children. First, how parents were raised shapes their beliefs and values about families, and their responsiveness to the needs of others.

Second, children's own characteristics contribute to how they are parented. An infant with a difficult temperament may strain immature parents, who may become hostile toward their baby.

Third, parents have sources of support and stress in relationships with family, friends, and work. A mutually supportive marital relationship is the foundation for raising a healthy child, whereas a troubled marriage undermines child development. Family and friends can provide child care, advice, and emotional support, but they can also be intrusive. Around the world, parents have the same hierarchy of goals for their children. They want them to be safe and healthy, to grow up to support themselves and their own families, and to share the values of the family and community (**Part A**).

39 Homeless Children

Homeless children

The typical homeless person in America is a child.

Children and families make up the fastest-growing segment of the homeless population.

The typical homeless family is a single, 20-year-old mother with 2 children under the age of 6.

Over one-third of homeless families have an open case for child abuse or neglect. One out of 5 has lost at least 1 child to foster care.

Nearly half of homeless children either have witnessed or have been subjected to violence in their homes.

Over half of all homeless children never have lived in their own home. Over 40% have been homeless more than once.

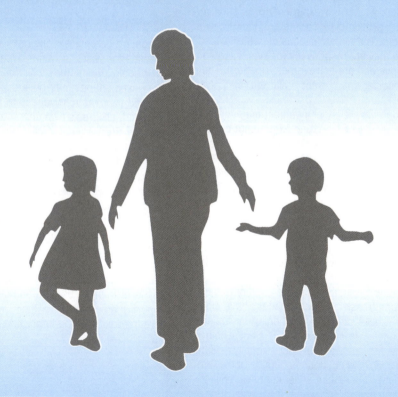

Today *homeless* refers to those who rely on shelters for their residence, or who live on the streets or in parks. They are not just alcoholic men clustered together on skid rows. The new homeless population is younger and much more mixed: more single women, more families, and more minorities. The **Table** presents facts on homelessness. Nationally, families with children are the fastest-growing segment of the homeless population, constituting about 40%.

Who Are the Homeless?

On any given night, 100,000 children in this country are homeless (Walsh, 1992). They are also characterized by few social contacts, poor health, and a high level of contact with the criminal justice system. The typical homeless family of modern American society consists of an unmarried 20-year-old mother with 1 or 2 children under the age of 6 years, probably fathered by different men.

Homeless families are forced to move frequently: Length-of-stay restrictions in shelters, short stays with relatives and friends, and relocation to seek employment make it difficult for children to have any sense of stability. Their health suffers, any sense of security is minimal, and schooling is almost nonexistent. Even when school is available, children often lack the means to attend because of a lack of transportation.

Consequently, it would be a mistake to think of homelessness as merely a housing problem. It is an educational issue, a children's issue, and a family issue, and if all of these issues are not addressed, remedial efforts are destined to fail.

The Impact of Homelessness on Development

Homeless children, like all people, have different levels of stress tolerance. The causes of homelessness, the length of time without a home, the availability of (or lack of) support systems, and the age, sex, and temperament of children all produce different reactions. Feelings of depression, anxiety, and low self-esteem are frequent accompaniments and often lead to either aggression or withdrawal. Truancy, hyperactivity, and underachievement are no strangers to these children. Here are several specific difficulties the homeless experience (Dacey and Travers, 1999).

Health

Homeless individuals experience illness and injury much more than the general population does. Health care is lacking because they do not have health insurance; thus, homeless children have much higher rates of acute and chronic health problems. Homeless women have significantly more LBW babies and higher levels of infant mortality. Homeless children are more susceptible to asthma, ear infections, and diarrhea and are less likely to receive recommended immunizations on schedule.

Hunger and Poor Nutrition

Homeless families struggle to maintain an adequate and nutritionally balanced diet in the setting of no refrigerator, no stove, poor food, and lack of food. Homeless children and their families often depend on emergency food assistance. Many times the facilities themselves suffer from a lack of resources, with the result that the children, and their families, go hungry.

Developmental Delays

Homeless children experience, to a significantly higher degree than typical children, motor coordination difficulties, language delays, cognitive delays, social inadequacies, and a lack of personal skills (e.g., do not know how to eat at a table). The instability of their lives, the disruptions in child care, an erratic pattern of schooling, and how parents adapt to these conditions also impede development.

Psychological Problems

Homeless children seem to suffer more than typical children from depression, anxiety, and behavioral problems. Data that might enable identification of the particular aspect of homelessness that causes a child's anxiety or depression are lacking. But parental depression affects children, and their children's problems may reflect the parents' own feeling of helplessness.

Educational Underachievement

Homeless children do poorly in reading and mathematics. This finding should come as no surprise, given that these children have difficulty in finding and maintaining free public education for substantial periods. These children also miss the remedial work they so urgently need.

Schools are now mandated to provide school services that are comparable to those other children receive. In 1990, the act was amended to ensure that all homeless children are provided adequate transportation to school, are placed on an immunization schedule, and are furnished their school and health records and that guardianship requirements are met.

Implications for Health Care Providers

You may encounter homeless children in a number of ways, often in the emergency room, where homeless families go for their primary care. These children frequently come to the attention of school nurses who may discover mental or physical disabilities. Today, nurses are more evident in shelters and other agencies that serve the homeless, doing health teaching and routine screenings to identify health problems.

40 Divorce

A Children of divorce

Year	Marriages	Rate/1,000	Divorces	Rate/1,000
1920	1,274,000	12.0	171,000	1.6
1930	1,127,000	9.2	196,000	1.6
1940	1,596,000	12.1	264,000	2.0
1950	1,667,000	11.1	385,000	2.6
1960	1,523,000	8.5	393,000	2.2
1970	2,163,000	10.6	708,000	3.5
1980	2,390,000	10.0	1,036,000	4.8
1990	2,448,000	9.8	1,175,000	4.7
1996	2,344,000	8.8	1,150,000	4.3

B Living arrangements of children under 18 years old (in thousands)

Arrangement:	1970	1980	1990	1995
Living with 2 parents	58,939 (85.2%)	48,624 (76.7%)	46,503 (72.5%)	48,276 (68.7%)
1 Parent	8,199 (11.9%)	12,466 (19.7%)	15,867 (24.7%)	18,938 (27.0%)
Mother	7,452 (10.8%)	11,406 (18.0%)	13,874 (21.6%)	16,477 (23.4%)
Father	748 (1.1%)	1,060 (1.7%)	1,993 (3.1%)	2,461 (3.5%)
Relatives	1,547 (2.2%)	1,949 (3.1%)	1,421 (2.2%)	2,352 (3.3%)
Nonrelatives	477 (0.7%)	388 (0.6%)	346 (0.5%)	688 (1.0%)

The following statistics tell the story, starkly and unrelentingly: Nearly half of today's marriages will end in divorce and an estimated 50% of children will live with a single parent before the age of 18. Although the divorce rate has remained stable (but still high) over the past decade (see **Part A**), the United States has a larger number of single parents than any other developed country.

Children and Divorce

Children of divorce and separation face multiple transitions in their lives. They experience the shock of the initial separation and often a move to new living conditions—new housing, new school, new friends. Simultaneously, they typically are involved in a visitation schedule, perhaps 1 weekend a month, with the separated parent. Since most divorced adults remarry, the cycle is repeated: the transition to another new home, a strange adult, any children of the new adult, and new adjustments to schools, teachers, and friends. Children from divorced and remarried families tend to exhibit more behavioral problems and are less academically, socially, and psychologically well adjusted than those in nondivorced families. However, 70%–80% of children from divorced families do not show severe or enduring problems in their reactions to their parents' marital changes. They develop as reasonably competent and well-adjusted individuals (Hetherington and Stanley-Hagen, 1995). **Part B** provides data on the living arrangements of children under 18 years old.

Children's Reactions to Divorce

Young childrens' ability to engage in abstract thinking is still limited and they still cannot reverse their thinking, which colors their reaction to their parents' divorce. For example, they may think that *they* are responsible. Consequently, parents about to divorce should explain the reasons for the divorce to their children in a manner and terms that match the children's ability to understand.

Children's Adjustment to Divorce

Following the divorce, it takes most children about 2 or 3 years to adjust to living in a single-parent home. This adjustment, however, can once again be shaken when a parent remarries. It means losing 1 parent in the divorce, adapting to life with the remaining parent, and the addition of at least 1 new member in a remarriage.

The transition period in the first year following the divorce is stressful economically, socially, and emotionally. Conditions then seem to improve, and children in a stable, smoothly functioning home are better adjusted than children in a nuclear family riddled with conflict. Nevertheless, school achievement may suffer and impulsivity may increase (Dacey and Travers, 1999).

A well-known student of the effects of divorce on children, Judith Wallerstein (1983) identified several psychological tasks that children face in adjusting to their parents' divorce.

1. **Facing the reality of the divorce.** This task relates to a child's cognitive level. Young children simply cannot understand the complexities surrounding their parents' marital rupture, and even older children may at first deny it. Although children come to accept the fact of the split, some still dream about their parents reuniting. For example, Wallerstein and Blakeslee (1989) reported what they termed *reconciliation fantasies.* Ten years after their parents' divorce, and even after remarriage, some children hope their parents can get together again.
2. **Resuming their own daily lives.** Initially, children may be overwhelmed by what is happening around them. Their schoolwork, their play, and their relationships reflect the fallout from their concern about their parents. They gradually adjust and immerse themselves in their daily lives.
3. **Reconciling themselves to loss.** A way of life changes and, with the separation of a parent, children frequently experience a loss of security. Their world has been severely shaken; some children come to adjust, whereas others find it difficult to fully regain their equilibrium.
4. **Dealing with their emotions.** Some children never really forgive their parents (or parent) and build a reservoir of anger that affects their lives for years. Many of their actions as adolescents, and even adults, reflect the anger that they have carried with them from the time of the divorce. Resolving these feelings is a critical task for healthy adult adjustment.
5. **Developing a positive outlook for the future.** Children often avoid any close relationship because of their fear of desertion. Most children regain their sense of trust in others, but some experience continuing problems in maintaining relationships.

Implications for Health Care Providers

In your work with children, you'll inevitably find those who are experiencing the shock of family conflict. The behavioral and emotional repercussions affect every aspect of their lives—friendships, schoolwork, and even health. When you contact these children, be alert to emotional issues: illness, aggression (or withdrawal), irritability, and so on. Try to attain a comfortable closeness with them so that they realize you are a trusted "secure base."

If at all possible, work with parents and encourage them to keep their children's needs in focus, not an easy task given their personal emotional crisis. Most parents recognize that they themselves must be, as much as possible, a source of consistent support for their children. Your task, then, is to help parents reach this conclusion, while you offer as much waarmth and security as possible for the children.

41 Day Care

A Federal agency requirements for day care

1. Planned activities that are developmentally appropriate and that promote children's intellectual, social, emotional, and physical development.
2. Caregivers with specialized training, especially regarding health and safety standards.
3. Nutritious meals.
4. A health record for each child.
5. Opportunities for parents to observe and to discuss their child's needs.
6. Small group sizes and low child-staff ratios.

B Characteristics of high-quality day care for preschool children

Program Characteristics	Signs of Quality
Physical setting	Indoor environment is clean, in good repair, well-ventilated. Classroom space is divided into richly equipped activity areas: make-believe play, blocks, science, math, games, puzzles, art, books, music. Fenced outdoor play area has swings, climbing equipment, tricycles, sandbox.
Group size	No more than 18–20 students with 2 teachers.
Child-caregiver ratio	Ratio of 8 children to 1 caregiver in centers; 6 to 1 in family day care.
Daily activities	Children work individually and/or in small groups, selecting their own activities. Caregivers facilitate children's involvement, adjusting expectations to fit the child.
Teacher qualifications	Caregivers have college-level specialized preparation in early childhood development, education, or related field.
Relationships with parents	Parents are encouraged to be involved, to observe, to meet with caregivers to discuss child's development.
Licensing/accreditation	Program is licensed by state. Centers and preschool programs are accredited by National Academy of Early Childhood Programs. Family day care is accredited by National Association for Family Day Care.

After World War II, middle-class families could afford to have 1 parent at home full-time, an unprecedented economic luxury. By 1968, 35% of mothers with children ages 3–5 were working. Today, 65% of mothers with children under age 6 work outside of the home, leaving their children in someone else's care (Shonkoff, 1995). Parents' choice of a day care setting for their children is limited by availability, cost, and quality.

Day Care Settings

Some children are cared for in their own homes by either a relative or nonrelative. Family day care is provided in someone else's home. Day care centers are located in churches, parents' workplaces, and the community. Many children are cared for in more than 1 setting; for example, they spend the morning at a center and the afternoon with a grandparent.

Of all children under 5 years, 35.6% are in family day care, 30% are cared for in their own homes, and 24% are in day care centers. Among children ages 3–6, these percentages are 17%, 18%, and 43%, respectively (U.S. Census Bureau, 1988). Preschoolers are more likely to be cared for in day care centers because many centers double as nursery schools. The older the child is at the time of entry to day care, the more likely the child is to be placed in a day care center.

Developmental Effects of Day Care

There has been considerable concern that nonparent child care can disrupt attachment between mother and child, or have a negative impact on social development. Others counter that for disadvantaged children, day care can be a form of early intervention, providing an enriching environment when one does not exist at home.

The implications of day care for development include many factors: how many day care settings the child has experienced, how many hours the child is in day care, the quality and stability of the care, the type of setting, and the child's age at entry. A child's day care experience must be examined in light of the characteristics of individual children, such as gender and temperament, and their families, especially socioeconomic status and parenting behaviors.

Day Care and Attachment
The National Institute of Child Health and Development (NICHD) examines the effects of day care on over a thousand children at 10 different sites. Results indicate that children who have been in day care are no different from those cared for by their mothers in regards to mother-child attachment, as measured using the "strange situation" technique (see Chapter 29).

The best direct predictors of attachment were not the type, quality, or amount of day care but psychological adjustment of the mother and mothering behavior. The more sensitive and responsive the mother is, the more likely a secure attachment will develop, regardless of whether or not a child has been in day care.

When low maternal sensitivity is combined with long hours of poor-quality day care, children, especially boys, are more likely to be insecurely attached or avoidant. These children have a "dual risk"; that is, poor-quality care at home and at day care undermines the development of secure attachment. For some children, high-quality day care may compensate for less-sensitive mothering. But poor-quality care does not necessarily undermine the development of a secure attachment if the mother is sensitive and responsive in her interactions with her child (NICHD, 1997).

Day Care and Social Development
Follow-up with the NICHD study of children at age 3 indicates that the incidence of behavior problems is also not related to whether or not a child is in day care, or how long a child has been in day care (NICHD, in press). Once again, mothering behaviors and characteristics are stronger predictors of child outcomes than is a child's day care experience per se. The quality of day care does matter. Children who have experienced higher-quality day care during their first 2 years have fewer behavior problems and are more compliant with adult direction (e.g., to help clean up) than are children who were cared for in lower-quality settings.

Quality of Care
NICHD noted that quality of day care is frequently higher for children from families with more economic advantages. Working mothers who are well adjusted, like their jobs, and have choices regarding day care are more likely to be sensitive and responsive when interacting with their children.

The United States lags far behind Western Europe in its attitude and policies regarding day care. Although there are federal requirements for day care (see **Part A**) (Clarke-Stewart, 1992), state requirements vary widely. NICHD found that quality of care seems to be improving since the first studies were done 15–20 years ago, perhaps because parents are more attuned to the issues involved. **Part B** lists characteristics of high-quality day care settings (National Association for the Education of Young Children, 1991).

42 Development of Self

A Key terms

Self-concept: the attributes, abilities, attitudes, and values by which one defines who he or she is

Self-esteem: aspect of self-concept that involves evaluations about one's worth

Self-regulation: ability to act in compliance with expectations using cues from parents

Self-control: ability to choose one's behavior and its consequences in accordance with acceptable norms and in the absence of authority figures

B Disciplinary strategies that support development of self-control

Strategy	Description	Example
Verbal instruction	Explain behavior.	"You can't just grab what you want. Next time, ask nicely."
Perspective taking	Provide other's point of view.	"It hurts when you hit her. You wouldn't want her to do that to you."
Role modeling	Adults demonstrate behavior.	Being quiet in church; talking through conflicts
Time-out	Remove child to quiet area. Set timer. Set contingency for return.	"Sit here for 5 minutes. When you're ready to play nicely, you can join us. Nicely means no grabbing."
Positive attribution	Verbally reward child.	"You were a big help. Thanks!"

C

Classic definition of self-esteem (William James, 1890)

$$\text{Self-esteem} = \frac{\text{Success}}{\text{Pretense}}$$

A sense of self is a multifaceted composite of one's characteristics and abilities (see **Part A**). Self-concept develops as children mature physically, cognitively, and socially, and is subject to influence from parents, peers, and society at large.

Self-recognition

A clever study suggested that children recognize themselves in a mirror by age 15 months (Lewis and Brooks-Gunn, 1979). While wiping a child's nose, researchers smudged it with rouge. Younger infants reached out to touch the nose in the mirror, whereas toddlers between 15 and 24 months responded to the image by wiping their own noses. Between ages 2 and 3, the growth of language and representational thought enables children to identify themselves in a picture and refer to themselves by name. They classify themselves using salient features, for example, boy, girl, big, little.

Agency and Self-regulation

As toddlers explore the world on their own terms, they develop a sense of agency: "I did it!" Parental expectations about what they should and should not do conflict with toddlers' desires. As a result, an emerging sense of agency is tempered by regulating one's own behavior in response to parental cues. Whereas a parent may need to physically remove a sharp object from a young toddler's reach, a word of caution about picking it up should suffice with a 3-year-old. Agency and self-regulation contribute to self-concept as children identify who they are by what they do.

Self-control

Self-regulation in response to parental cues must give way to self-control in the absence of authority figures. Children must understand the requirements of social situations, monitor their own behavior, and be motivated to exercise self-control. They also must understand the consequences of their behavior.

Many processes contribute to the development of self-control, such as being quiet in church. Preschoolers get better at regulating their verbal and physical impulses, especially when parents provide explanations ("we're here to listen"), reminders (a disapproving look), or diversions (a book to read), and model the desired behavior. Children internalize these processes, and remind themselves either out loud or in their heads about what is expected when parents are absent. Children do not learn self-control by themselves, and it develops over time.

Mastery over Aggressive Impulses

Children must learn to control their feelings and impulses. When toddlers experience overwhelming arousal, they throw a tantrum. Instrumental aggression appears as they push, pull, and grab to get their way. Young children have difficulty differentiating between "sad," "mad," and "bad" because they experience all of these when their intentions are thwarted by disapproving parents. They cry and strike out and try to hide, all at the same time. Hostile aggression, which is meant to hurt, increases between ages 4 and 7. At first it is physical, but as children hone their language skills, verbal insults and taunts increase. The goal is domination, but children learn that victory does not win friends.

Parents employ several disciplinary strategies to teach children to control their aggressive impulses (see **Part B**). Verbal instruction encourages children to take the perspective of others and offers alternative behaviors: "It hurts when you push her. How would you feel if she did that to you? If you want the toy, you need to ask for it, not push." Role modeling provides long-term effects when combined with verbal instruction: "I'm so angry right now that I need to leave the room to calm down." Time-out can be an effective way of helping children regain self-control, but works well with verbal instruction: "Are you ready to play nicely?" Remember young children cannot tell time, and parents should set a timer. Physical punishment such as slapping may stop aggressive behavior immediately, but the behavior escalates later. It also does not teach children the acceptable alternative to their misbehavior.

Self-esteem and Self-concept

Self-esteem is an evaluation of one's self-concept and inherent worth. During the preschool years, children's self-concept is categorical. It includes descriptions of clothing and hair color and names of siblings and pets. They refer to abilities, likes and dislikes, and emotions: "I can swim." "I like to play house." "I get mad." Preschool children can distinguish between how well others like them (social acceptance) from how well they can do something (competence): "Sara likes me, she's my friend." "I'm good at coloring."

By age 8, children have a general sense of self-esteem that is subdivided into academic, social, and physical components (Harter, 1990). With maturity, these become more complex: math versus English, sports versus appearance, and so on. School-age children are better judges of their abilities compared to peers than are preschool-age children. Ask a nursery school class who is the fastest runner, and all hands may go up. Ask a group of third graders, and there is a pause: Do you mean girl or boy? Do you mean in soccer or baseball?

Preschool children do not have either a general or a subdivided sense of self-esteem like their older siblings. Rather, they have an array of self-esteems depending on their experiences. For a 4-year-old, feeling good is the measure of success. Older children look at effort and outcome, and use information from several sources to evaluate themselves.

William James (1890), an American psychologist and philosopher, defined self-esteem as success divided by pretense (**Part C**). He conceptualized success as being fully human and real, as experiencing one's self as capable and as influencing events. Pretense means a self based on appearances, and lacking substance.

Gender development

Gender identity: categorizing one's self as either male or female (ages 2–3)

Gender constancy: understanding that one will always be the gender one is at present (ages 5–6)

Gender role: culturally accepted behavior based on gender, e.g.," mother" (appears by age 4 and evolves throughout life)

Gender stereotype: behavior that reflects characteristics commonly associated with being male or female, e.g., being aggressive vs being passive (by age 4)

Gender schema: theory that maintains gender is a social construction by which people organize information about what it means to be male or female in a given social order

Ambiguous genitals: genitalia that at birth are not clearly differentiated or fully developed as male or female due to chromosomal or hormonal aberrations

Oedipus complex: Freud's explanation of sexual identity in boys

Relational self: explanation by the Stone Center theorists of how girls develop a self

Rough and tumble play: interactions among peers involving friendly chasing, wrestling, and fighting that children recognize as pretend fun

Aggression: behavior that is intended to harm another person

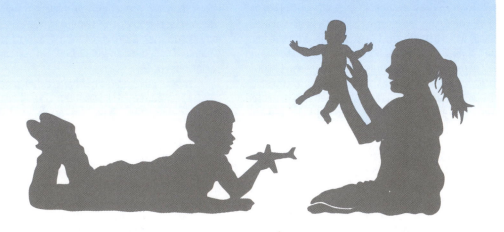

Gender development is multifaceted, occurs over a period of time, and has biological, social, and psychological influences (see **Part A**). It includes the ability to label one's self and others as male or female (gender identity), knowledge of gender roles, adoption of gender roles, and gender constancy, that is, recognizing that one's own gender is permanent. Cognitive-developmental theorists take the view that changes in cognitive ability and language combined with children's innate tendency to search the environment for cues about how to behave account for the development of gender knowledge and constancy. Social learning theory is associated with adoption of gender roles, that is, developing a preference for clothing and activities appropriate for one's own gender based on social experiences.

Gender schema theory attempts to reconcile the 2 theories. It maintains that gender is a social construction. That is, as a schema, gender is a way to organize information about the association between culture and gender. Gender schema includes what is considered masculine and feminine, the functional importance of gender in the social order, and the implications for concept of self as male or female.

Ages 2–3: Gender Labeling and Knowledge

Beginning at birth, adults respond differently to male and female infants; men and women treat infants differently as well. Men play more vigorously with babies, especially boys, whereas women talk to infants more, especially girls. By the age of 12 months, infants respond differently to pictures of male and female faces, suggesting they expect different types of interactions from men and women.

Toddlers begin to recognize themselves as individuals separate from their parents during the second year of life. Initially, concepts of self and gender are almost inseparable. A young toddler does not appreciate the anatomical differences between male and female, or that gender is 1 aspect of self.

By age 2½, children identify themselves as "boy" or "girl." After the second birthday, there is an increased expectation on the part of adults that young children learn to control their bodily functions. Because toilet training occurs at the same time as representational thinking and advances in language development, children can name body parts and their functions, communicate bodily urges to parents, and begin to anticipate their needs. Adults typically reward young children using gender-based language: "What a big boy you are!" "Aren't you a good girl!"

Gender identity is more than recognizing body parts. Between ages 2 and 3, children get better at labeling strangers as boys or girls, mommies or daddies, despite the fact that these individuals are fully clothed. Clearly children use social information about appearance and behavior to develop and label 2 categories of human beings.

Ages 3–5: Gender Constancy and Role

Between ages 3 and 5, children's knowledge about gender roles and stereotypes becomes more complete and complex. They still may have difficulty with gender constancy. Cognitive-developmental theorists explain this as an inability to conserve gender, that is, to recognize that it remains the same despite alterations in outward appearances.

Bem (1985) attributes this difficulty to gender schema. She relates the story of the day her son Jeremy decided to wear barrettes to nursery school. Another boy insisted that Jeremy was a girl because "only girls wear barrettes." When Jeremy pulled down his pants as proof, the other boy dismissed the physical evidence by proclaiming that "everybody has a penis but only girls wear barrettes." According to Bem, the social construction of gender is more powerful than anatomy.

During the preschool period, children recognize that to fit the category "male" or "female," they have to look and behave the part. Sex-typed behavior increases by age 4 as children become very rigid in their views of gender roles. It is as if by adhering to stereotyped behavior, they can assure themselves of gender identity and constancy. "Boys do this, I do this, so I am a boy." By ages 5–6, most children appreciate that gender is a permanent aspect of one's self-identity.

Rigidity regarding gender roles is in part attributable to a lack of cognitive flexibility. Recall that preschoolers focus on 1 aspect of something at a time, and are unable to coordinate multiple pieces of information. Also, parenting style, cultural influences, and children's emotional investment in gender roles contribute to their adoption of stereotyped behaviors. Children, especially boys, value the gender role of their own sex more highly.

Despite concern about unfair feminine stereotypes, boys may be more rigidly socialized into their gender role than girls. For example, a girl who plays with trucks is still more acceptable than a boy who plays with dolls. Only 15% of boys truly fit the picture of the "rough and tumble" boy (about 5%–7% of girls do), yet physically aggressive behavior has been expected and endorsed in boys throughout the ages: "Now of all wild young things a boy is the most difficult to handle . . . he is the craftiest, most mischievous, and unruliest of brutes" (Plato 427–347 BC).

Gender development

Gender identity: categorizing one's self as either male or female (ages 2–3)

Gender constancy: understanding that one will always be the gender one is at present (ages 5–6)

Gender role: culturally accepted behavior based on gender, e.g.," mother" (appears by age 4 and evolves throughout life)

Gender stereotype: behavior that reflects characteristics commonly associated with being male or female, e.g., being aggressive vs being passive (by age 4)

Gender schema: theory that maintains gender is a social construction by which people organize information about what it means to be male or female in a given social order

Ambiguous genitals: genitalia that at birth are not clearly differentiated or fully developed as male or female due to chromosomal or hormonal aberrations

Oedipus complex: Freud's explanation of sexual identity in boys

Relational self: explanation by the Stone Center theorists of how girls develop a self

Rough and tumble play: interactions among peers involving friendly chasing, wrestling, and fighting that children recognize as pretend fun

Aggression: behavior that is intended to harm another person

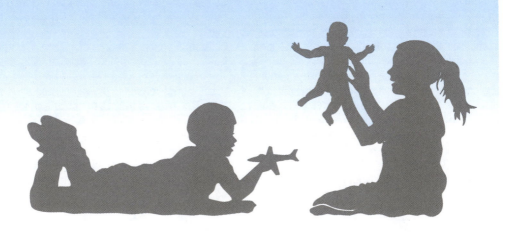

Psychodynamic Explanations of Gender Development

Freud's "Oedipus complex" refers to the small boy's need to separate "male self" from "female mother" and yet still retain "female" as an object of sexual desire. Freud thought that boys could accomplish this by competing with their fathers for the mother's affection. By defeating the father with whom they identified, boys secured their sexual identity. Cross-cultural research reveals the competition can be with a father figure (e.g., an uncle or older brother), suggesting that a boy is testing himself against the cultural power structure into which he is being socialized.

Freud's attempts to explain the corollary "Electra complex" in girls were inadequate. While little girls may express a desire to marry their father and get rid of their mother, they must continue to identify with their mother's gender role. That is, in Freud's view, girls are left to identify with the vanquished. Researchers at the Stone Center at Wellesley College, unlike Freud, believe women's sense of self is based on relationships with others, not on being separate from them. In forming a self, a young girl differentiates, not separates, her femaleness from that of her mother.

Biology and Gender

The relationship between biology and gender is more complex than previously thought. For example, genetic males (XY) who were insensitive to male hormones (androgens) prenatally are born with ambiguous genitals, which may be surgically corrected to be female. John Money (Money and Ehrhardt, 1972) initially found that when these children were raised as girls, they developed female gender role behaviors, including sexual orientation. Money concluded that gender identity is a product of social rearing and not genetics or biology. Recent research suggests that the development of gender identity and sexual orientation is not so easily assigned by rearing alone. During adolescence, some individuals who have surgically corrected genitals or who are hermaphrodites have requested that their gender identity be reassigned to the sex opposite their rearing (Diamond, 1997). Clearly, the relationships between chromosomes, hormones, brain development, and socialization are still not well understood.

Aggression is another example. While rough and tumble play is more common among boys than girls, the difference is not easily attributed to biology. Early research suggested that girls exposed to elevated levels of male hormones prenatally had been masculinized, that is, exhibited more tomboy behavior. Follow-up studies suggest the definition of "tomboy" may have been biased, and that the girls are happy being girls. Also contrary to popular belief, males with XYY chromosomes are not more aggressive than XY males (Dabbs, 1992). Rough and tumble play among both girls and boys is not the same thing as aggression, nor does it lead to aggression. Both appear to be cultural, not biological, phenomena.

45 **Play Behavior**

Play

Play Type	Age (yr)	Definition	Examples
Sensorimotor play	0–2	Plays using body	Kicking crib
Pretend play	0–6	Play shifts from solitary to social	Pretend gestures; imitating parents' roles
Functional play	1–2	Simple, repetitive motor movements with or without objects	Running around, rolling a toy car back and forth
Constructive play	3–6	Creating or constructing something	Making a house out of toy blocks, drawing a picture, putting a puzzle together
Make-believe play	3–7	Acting out roles	Playing house, school, or doctor; acting as a television character
Games with rules	6–11	Understanding and following rules in games	Playing board games, cards, baseball, etc.

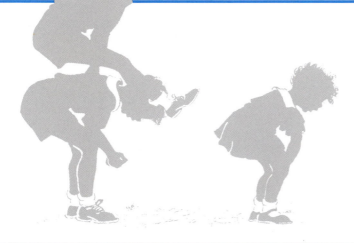

Children cherish their play. Shouting, running, chasing each other, enjoying games, engaging in make-believe, and exploring their worlds, children love to have fun.

During early childhood, children engage their world symbolically: letting one thing represent another, adopting different types of roles, and indulging in fantasy and pretend activities. Children may pretend to drink from play cups, or feed a doll with a spoon, or pretend a box is a truck. Pretend play is a major characteristic of this developmental period. Play also becomes more social, and interactions with other children become more important.

Defining Play

Several key elements of play contribute to its definition:

- Play must be enjoyable and valued by the player.
- Play has no extrinsic goals; that is, play is intrinsically motivated.
- Play is spontaneous and voluntary; no one is forcing children to play; they freely choose it.
- Play demands that children be actively engaged.
- Play has systematic relations to other behavior that is not play (Garvey, 1990).

Let's define *play* as an activity that children engage in because they enjoy it for its own sake. Children play in a wide variety of situations: alone or with others, with objects, and with ideas. Children's play may be simple, but it also demonstrates great skill and dexterity in complicated patterns.

Explanations of Play

In his book *Play, Dreams, and Imitation in Childhood* (1962), Piaget stated that children initially use their physical activities to build their cognitive structures (see Chapter 3). When children continue these physical acts for the amusement in them, however, Piaget believed they were playing. Sooner or later children grasp for the pleasure of grasping, and swing for the sake of swinging.

Piaget next turned his attention to the games children play, identifying 3 types: practice games, symbolic games, and games with rules. Each of these games matches the major stages of cognitive development. During early childhood, symbolic games aid children's development by reproducing their world.

Another, and quite different explanation of play can be found in psychoanalytic theory (see Chapter 1). Freud believed that play provided children with a means for wish fulfillment and a way to overcome the traumatic events in their lives. It allows children to escape the restrictions of reality and permits them to rid themselves of dangerous, aggressive impulses. Play also supports children's desire to imitate those they love and admire, thus fulfilling the wish to be like these models.

Mastery of the traumatic events of their lives occurs through *repetition compulsion*. Inevitably children will have experiences that they find too intense to assimilate psychologically. In their play, then, children repeat elements of the disturbing event and gradually diminish the intensity of the initial experience, leading to feelings of mastery.

Erikson (see Chapter 2) believed that the form play takes changes as a child's psychosocial issues change. For the most part, children struggle to make sense of their world and bring it under control. For Erikson, games can be just fun, but they can also be an occasion of social sharing as well as a means of working out an emotional problem.

Play's Contributions to Development

Physical Development

Children play for the sheer exuberance of it; play enables them to exercise their bodies and improve motor skills. The physical activities of running, throwing, and kicking, for example, contribute to children's health, strength, and endurance. When they start to throw and catch a ball, the benefits of muscular coordination and eye-hand coordination are obvious, and they continue to develop feelings of mastery of their environment.

Cognitive Development

Beginning with the notion that play has widespread consequences, we can say that play allows children to explore their environment on their own terms and to take in any meaningful experiences at their own rate and on their own level (e.g., running through a field and stopping to look at rocks or insects). Consequently, play aids cognitive development and cognitive development aids play.

Social Development

Play helps social development during this period because the involvement of others demands a give-and-take that teaches young children the basics of forming relationships. Social skills demand the same building processes as cognitive skills. These social skills do not simply appear; they are learned and much of the learning comes through play (Dacey and Travers, 1999).

Implications for Health Care Providers

When you come in contact with children, they are probably uncertain, frightened, and anxious, which is why health care settings have become more child friendly. The use of playrooms in hospitals, where examinations, shots, and changing of dressings are not permitted, reflects the attempt to reduce children's anxiety. One way of easing their anxiety is to engage in some type of game—playing with toys, pretend, or a board game they're familiar with. Let them choose whatever they want and use the opportunity to ease them into a more accepting attitude.

PART IV: QUESTIONS

Directions: For each of the following questions, choose the **one best** answer.

1. You are going down the stairs behind a little boy who is placing both feet on each step as he goes while holding the railing. About how old is he?

(A) 3 years old

(B) 4 years old

(C) 5 years old

(D) 6 years old

2. What skill that is essential for reading readiness develops between ages 3 and 6?

(A) Using hands as tools

(B) Coping and tracing figures

(C) Visuomotor scanning

(D) Recognizing the letters of the alphabet

3. You are pouring juice for a 4-year-old and 10-year-old into 2 different glasses, one short and wide, the other tall and narrow. The 4-year-old insists on having the tall narrow glass despite assurances from the 10-year-old that the 2 glasses have the same amount of juice. What term is used to describe the 4-year-old's understanding of this situation?

(A) Centration

(B) Appearance reality

(C) Cause by association

(D) Difficulty with conservation

4. Which of the following is an example of a child's difficulty with conservation during the preschool period?

(A) Thinks a ball of clay gets bigger when it is rolled into a snake

(B) Given 2 rows of M&Ms with 10 in each row, will say the row more spread out has more

(C) Says the glass with the most juice is the taller one, even if child just saw the juice poured from a shorter but wider glass

(D) All of the above

5. Montessori's ideas concerning _____ periods are important in planning preschool programs.

(A) lengthy

(B) class

(C) sensitive

(D) daily

6. Preschool educators are alert to match materials and methods to appropriate ages because of

(A) Piaget.

(B) Freud.

(C) Skinner.

(D) Pavlov.

7. The rules of _____ describe how to put words together to form sentences.

(A) phonology

(B) semantics

(C) grammar

(D) pragmatics

8. "Daddy *camed* home" is an example of

(A) overextension.

(B) mispronunciation.

(C) overregulation.

(D) delayed language.

9. Parents who value compliance with their authority and set nonnegotiable standards for their children's behavior are examples of which type of parenting, according to Baumrind?

(A) Authoritative

(B) Authoritarian

(C) Permissive

(D) Neglectful

10. Which of the following factors contribute to how parents parent?

(A) Childhood experiences of parents

(B) Personality characteristics of children being parented

(C) Work environment of parents, especially fathers

(D) All of the above

11. Which of the following conditions is not necessarily associated with homelessness?

(A) Health problems

(B) Hunger

(C) Poor nutrition

(D) Low intelligence

12. Recent additions to the number of homeless are

(A) mothers and young children.

(B) single fathers.

(C) those with alcohol problems.

(D) those with drug problems.

13. One of the major adjustments a child may experience following the divorce of parents is to

(A) siblings.

(B) transitions.

(C) relatives.

(D) synchronicity.

14. Even after their divorced parents remarry, some children still believe their natural parents will reunite. This is called

(A) hopeful planning.

(B) wishful thinking.

(C) reconciliation fantasies.

(D) psychic cognition.

15. Erikson called it the period of initiative versus guilt; that is, children recognize they choose and are responsible for their behavior. Plato referred to it as "a constitutional government within them." Freud thought the superego as "a garrison in the conquered city of the id" is similar. What developmental task of the preschool years are they referring to?

(A) Agency

(B) Sense of self

(C) Mastery of aggression

(D) Self-control

16. Which of the following is an example of a 4-year-old's concept of self?

(A) "I am a better swimmer than my brother."

(B) "People like me because I play fair."

(C) "I like to swim."

(D) "I am better at drawing than at coloring."

17. By what age have children typically developed gender identity?

(A) 18 months

(B) 2½ years

(C) 3 years

(D) 5 years

18. Preschoolers tend to engage in sex-typed behaviors, such as boys playing with trucks and girls playing with dolls. How do developmentalists explain this phenomenon?

(A) Males and females have inborn sex-typed tendencies.

(B) Preschoolers are rewarded for exhibiting sex-typed behaviors.

(C) Girls are more rigidly socialized to exhibit certain behaviors than are boys.

(D) Preschoolers are developing concepts of gender constancy and role.

19. The most common type of play during early childhood is _____ play.

(A) physical

(B) unrestricted

(C) social

(D) pretend

20. Children play for fun, learning, and

(A) emotional release.

(B) cognitive dissonance.

(C) physical alignment.

(D) social graces.

PART IV: ANSWERS AND EXPLANATIONS

1. The answer is A.

At age 3, children can go upstairs using alternating feet, but still descend placing both feet on each step. By age 4, they descend using alternating feet and holding the railing. At age 6, they are running up and down stairs easily.

2. The answer is C.

Vision is 20/20 by age 4. Children also become more efficient and proficient in how they move their eyes to scan a page, an ability essential for reading readiness. At age 3, when asked to find the little mouse on the page of a favorite book, children initially scan haphazardly, looking here and there. Systematic scanning side to side and up and down develops between ages 3 and 6.

3. The answer is A.

They focus on only 1 aspect of something at a time—often the most obvious aspect—and fail to consider how several aspects might interact to produce the event. When pouring juice between a tall skinny glass and a short wide glass, they focus on only the height of the tall skinny glass in concluding that it is "bigger" and so contains more juice. They cannot account for height and width simultaneously.

4. The answer is D.

Conservation refers to the ability to understand that something remains the same even if its appearance is altered and nothing was seen to be taken away or added. Because preschool children are swayed by appearances, focus on 1 aspect of something at a time, and have difficulty working out events in their minds, they have difficulty with conservation tasks, such as those related to number, quantity, mass, and length.

5. The answer is C.

Montessori firmly believed that at certain ages in children's lives they are more attuned or ready (sensitive) for certain experiences.

6. The answer is A.

Piaget's identification of cognitive stages contributed to a desire to "match the mix," that is, to make sure that appropriate material would be available for certain ages and stages.

7. The answer is C.

Syntax is how words are put together to make sentences. In their acquisition of language, children quickly learn the rules of language that enable them to express themselves in a sensible manner to other members of their culture.

8. The answer is C.

Since children are rule learners, they frequently stay with the rule, even when they know the correct form, which is the meaning of overregulation. This phase of language development is common and nothing to worry about.

9. The answer is B.

Authoritarian parents aim to control their children's behavior by enforcing absolute standards for behavior. They value unquestioned respect for and compliance with authority, and discourage verbal give-and-take with their children. Authoritarian parents resolve conflicts through power assertion; that is, they lay down the law "or else."

10. The answer is D.

Research identifies 3 factors that determine how people parent their children. First, how parents were raised during their own childhood shapes their beliefs and values about families. Second, children's own characteristics contribute to how they are parented. For example, an infant with a difficult temperament may strain immature parents, who may become hostile toward their baby. Third, parents have sources of support and stress in relationships with family, friends, and work. For example, fathers employed in subordinate positions in organizations with a hierarchical power structure tend to have an authoritarian style of parenting at home.

11. The answer is D.

A person's intelligence is not linked to conditions such as homelessness. This question points out, however, how easily we may jump to conclusions about surface features.

12. The answer is A.

An alarming statistic is the rising number of single mothers with young children in homeless shelters. There has long been a tendency to view those in shelters as having problems with alcohol, but the change in this population necessitates a change in strategies for dealing with this new group.

13. The answer is B.

Given the current divorce rate, and the rate of divorce following second marriages, children are often shifted from home to home, school to school, etc. These transitions require considerable parental sensitivity, which many parents, given their emotional state, find difficult.

14. The answer is C.

Research has shown that some children hold on to these fantasies for many years, testifying to the effects of divorce on children.

15. The answer is D.

Self-regulation in response to parental cues must give way to self-control in the absence of authority figures. Children must understand the requirements of social situations, monitor their own behavior, and be motivated to exercise self-control. They also must understand the consequences of their behavior. A moral conscience develops during these years.

16. The answer is C.

During the preschool years, children's self-concept is categorical. It includes descriptions of clothing and hair color, names of siblings and pets, their school, and prized possessions. They refer to abilities, likes and dislikes, and emotions: "I can swim." "I like to play house." "I get mad." Preschool children can distinguish between how well others like them (social acceptance) from how well they can do something (competence): "Sara likes me, she's my friend." "I'm good at coloring."

17. The answer is B.

By age 2½, children identify themselves as "boy" or "girl." Because toilet training occurs at the same time as representational thinking and advances in language development, children can name body parts and their functions, communicate bodily urges to parents, and begin to anticipate their needs. Gender identity is more than recognizing body parts. Between ages 2 and 3, children get better at labeling strangers as boys or girls, mommies or daddies, despite the fact that these individuals are fully clothed. Clearly children use social information about appearance and behavior to develop and label 2 categories of human beings.

18. The answer is D.

During the preschool period, children recognize that to fit the category "male" or "female," they have to look and behave the part. Sex-typed behavior increases by age 4 as children become very rigid in their views of gender roles. It is as if by adhering to stereotyped behavior, they can assure themselves of gender identity and constancy. "Boys do this, I do this, so I am a boy." By ages 5–6, most children appreciate that gender is a permanent aspect of one's self-identity. Rigidity regarding gender roles is in part attributable to a lack of cognitive flexibility. Recall that preschoolers focus on 1 aspect of something at a time, and are unable to coordinate multiple pieces of information. Also, parenting style, cultural influences, and children's emotional investment in gender roles contribute to their adoption of stereotyped behaviors.

19. The answer is D.

Pretend play fits well with the growing cognitive ability during early childhood. Although all types of play are attractive, pretend play is particularly prominent during these years.

20. The answer is A.

Play allows children to release emotional tensions that they may not be allowed to express in school or home, a form of childhood therapy that furthers development.

PART V
Middle Childhood

46 Growth and Development

A Average vital statistics

Age (yr)	Boys Ht. (cm)	Boys Wt. (kg)	Girls Ht. (cm)	Girls Wt. (kg)	Resting Pulse (bpm)	Blood Pressure (mm Hg)
7	121	22.8	120.6	21.8	75–115	97/56
8	127	25.3	126.4	24.8	70–110	99/60
9	132	28	132	28.5	70–110	101/61
10	137	31.4	138.2	32.5	65–100	102/62
11	143	35.3	144.8	40	60–100	105/63
12	150	40	151.5	41.5	55–90	107/64

B Physical development

Age (yr)	Gross/Fine Motor	General Physical	Adaptive Skills
7	Rides 2-wheel bike More cautious Prints well Copies diamond	Average height: 120–122 cm Average weight: 21–23 kg Begins to grow 5 cm/yr Incisors erupting	Brushes and combs hair Uses table knife to cut, may need help Reads face clock
8–9	Movement fluid, graceful, limber Always on the go Hard to quiet down Smoother fine movements Uses cursive writing	Average height: 127–132 cm Average weight: 24–28 kg Still grows 5 cm/yr Jaw grows to accommodate permanent teeth	Uses common tools: saw, hammer, screwdriver Helps with household tasks: sweeping Runs useful errands
10–12	Active in physical sports Can break a physical skill into individual steps Practices physical skills Uses keyboard	Boys: slow growth in height but rapid weight gain Girls: taller than boys, pubescent changes Remainder of permanent teeth erupt; braces?	Cooks and sews a bit Does easy repair work Can be responsible for chores, with reminders Can be left alone for an hour or so

Growth in height and weight is slower and steadier during middle childhood (ages 7–12) than the preschool years. Differences between boys and girls are minimal until ages 10–12 when girls grow taller than boys, and boys put on extra weight but not height. Girls also begin to experience pubertal changes (see Chapter 53); the average age of menarche for American girls is 12 years. For boys, puberty arrives at about age 14.

Organ systems become more efficient and adult-like. As the gastrointestinal system matures and grows in capacity, children experience fewer stomachaches, can go longer between meals, and require fewer calories. Heart and respiratory rates decline as blood pressure increases between ages 6 and 12. The organization of the central nervous system (CNS) is like an adult's, although the frontal lobes, the site of reasoning ability, continue to mature.

Body proportions also change. Children have a lower center of gravity. There is an increase in leg length, decrease in head size, and decrease in waist size relative to height. These slender proportions contribute to physical agility, so that riding a bike or hiking a mountain trail is better coordinated. There is an increase in muscle mass relative to body weight, although muscles are still immature and vulnerable to injuries from overuse. Bones continue to ossify, and if broken will heal more quickly than during adolescence because they are still growing.

Children start losing deciduous teeth at about age 6. They are replaced by permanent teeth by about age 12, with the exception of wisdom teeth which erupt later in adolescence. As the jaw grows to accommodate permanent adult-sized teeth, the mouth appears disproportionately large. As the eustachian tubes of the ears lengthen, they angle downward, allowing better drainage. Children experience fewer ear infections.

Middle childhood is often idealized as a period of rugged good health. Relatively secure in their agile bodies, children turn their attention outward. This is Erikson's period of industry, when children are busy developing physical, academic, and social skills. There are 2 key areas of health promotion for this age group: nutrition and injury prevention.

Nutrition and Obesity

Although caloric needs relative to body mass decrease during middle childhood, an average intake of 2,000 kcal/day is needed to sustain slow and steady growth. While very young children need fat and cholesterol in their diets to promote growth of the brain, school-age children do not. Their nutritional needs are best met using the food pyramid: grains, fresh fruits and vegetables, low-fat milk products, and lean meat and fish. Unfortunately, many American children consume too much fat and sugar, mostly in junk foods. Poor families use more high-fat, low-cost packaged foods, like mac-

aroni and cheese, and eat fewer fresh fruits and vegetables. According to the Children's Defense Fund, 12% of children in the United States are malnourished.

Malnourished American children tend to be obese, not thin. Obesity is defined as being 20% overweight for age, sex, and build due to excess accumulation of body fat; 27% of American children are obese. Other contributing factors are physical inactivity and family feeding practices. The average child who watches 4 hours of television a day is not playing outside, strengthening muscles and bones, and increasing aerobic capacity. Parents who overfeed children because they use food as reward and as solace, and who rush through meals, are more likely to raise obese children and be obese themselves. The pattern of inactivity and family habits that lead to obesity appear as early as 18 months.

Obesity represents a complex cycle of cause and consequence. Glucose metabolism in people who are obese favors the storage of fat but not its expenditure for energy. Children who are obese have more trouble sustaining physical activity and so avoid it, further isolating them socially. They soothe emotions using food, which adds to their weight and inactivity. Children who are fat report more depression and lower self-esteem than healthier peers. Obese children become obese teenagers. The best treatment involves the family and changing behaviors. Promoting healthy nutritional habits, exercise, and mutual support among family members is key.

Injury Prevention

The increased agility of school-age children combined with their maturing cognitive abilities (see Chapter 43) contributes to the decreased incidence of some injuries between ages 6 and 12 compared to the preschool years. Younger children are more likely to drown, fall from high places, and be scalded by hot water. Injuries remain the leading cause of death between ages 1 and 19, accounting for more deaths than all other diseases combined. About 25% of children require medical attention for an injury each year. Boys have more frequent and more serious injuries than girls, probably because boys engage in more risk-taking behavior.

Two types of injury are prevalent among school-age children: bicycle accidents and sports injuries. Health education programs promote bike safety, encouraging students to use helmets, learn the rules of the road, and keep their bikes in working condition. In sports, demands on young athletes to train earlier, longer, and harder have increased the incidence of overuse injuries. While an acute blow does obvious damage, the more common and subtle damage is from repetitive microtrauma to muscles and joints that are not fully developed. Stress fractures and little leaguer's elbow are examples. It is the responsibility of adults to help children be healthy and safe.

47 Cognitive Development

A Characteristics of concrete operations

Characteristics	Examples
Decreasing centration	How much juice a glass holds depends on both its height and its width.
Reversibility of a mental sequence	If 5 minus 2 equals 3, then 3 plus 2 equals 5.
Set identity	If you have not added or subtracted anything, the set remains the same.
Conservation of mass	A piece of clay remains the same mass whether it is rolled in a snake or clumped together.
Conservation of number	Ten M&Ms are 10 M&Ms whether they are arranged in 1 row or 2.
Hierarchical classification	If you have 3 spaniels and 2 retrievers, you have more dogs than spaniels.
Matrix classification	Baseball cards are sorted by team and field position.

B An experiment to test for conservation of liquid

Step 1: Present a child with 2 clear glass or plastic containers, A and B. Put an equal amount of colored water in each one, for example, 1 cup.

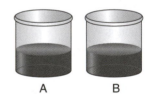

Step 2: Place a taller, thinner clear container, C, next to them. Now pour the contents of container B into C.

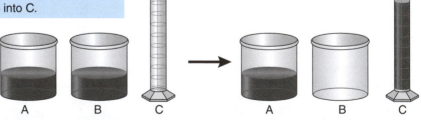

Step 3: Ask the child, "Which container has more colored water, A or C? Or do they both have the same amount of colored water? Why?" Let the child pour the colored water between the containers.

Characteristics of Concrete Operations

Between the ages of 5 and 7, an important shift takes place in how children organize information. Whereas the thinking of preschoolers is shaped by capricious influences, thinking in school-age children is determined by a logical internal organization. The shift is from associative to logical responding, from preoperational to concrete operational thinking. Logical thinkers love rules because rules organize experience and make life orderly.

In school-age children, concrete operational thinking consists of mental operations that allow children to do mentally what had to be experienced physically before. Actions can be played out in their minds, giving them more flexibility for solving problems. Concrete thought is characterized by decreasing centration, reversibility of a mental sequence, set identity, conservation of physical properties, classification skills, and an inability to think abstractly (see **Part A**).

Decreasing Centration

Decreasing centration refers to children's ability to consider 2 or more pieces of information at one time when solving a problem. Information can be held in and worked on in their mind. Concrete thinkers still need perceptual supports. They need to see the problem and to handle it physically in some way. A concrete thinker pouring juice into 2 different-sized glasses understands that how much juice a glass can hold depends on both its height and its width.

Reversibility of a Sequence

Concrete thinkers can think through a sequence of actions in their minds, and then reverse it to arrive back where they started. If 5 minus 2 equals 3, the operation can be reversed: 3 plus 2 equals 5. If you eat too much, you gain weight. If you eat less, you lose it. You can roll a ball of clay into a snake and then ball it up again.

Set Identity

Children understand that the identity of a set remains the same despite the fact that its physical properties are rearranged. They are not easily fooled by appearances. Ten M&Ms are still 10 M&Ms whether they are arranged in 1 row or 2. One piece of bread is still 1 piece of bread whether it is folded or cut up to make a sandwich.

Conservation of Physical Properties

Decreasing centration, reversibility of a sequence, and set identity contribute to a concrete thinker's ability to conserve physical properties. Children understand that some properties of an object remain the same even if they have acted on that object to alter its appearance. This understanding is the basis for science curricula.

When children understand that the 10 M&Ms are still 10 M&Ms, they are able to conserve number. Recognizing that the piece of clay is the same piece of clay no matter its shape is conservation of mass and length. Compensating for glasses of different heights and widths when pouring juice is conservation of quantity (see **Part B**). Knowing that a ton of feathers is the same as a ton of bricks is conservation of weight.

Classification Skills

Classification skills expand with the ability to engage in mental operations. *Hierarchical classification* refers to the ability to understand the relationship between subordinate and superordinate classes. Spaniels and retrievers are dogs. If the family has 3 spaniels and 2 retrievers, it has more dogs than spaniels. This understanding is the basis for addition and subtraction.

Matrix classification skills are more complex. Children can categorize things along 2 dimensions simultaneously, for example, color by type. A 2-by-2 matrix would consist of 2 rows of color (red and blue) and 2 columns of types (cars and blocks). Given a red car, school-age children will place it correctly in the matrix. This ability is needed to understand multiplication and division in math—and for sorting baseball cards.

Limitations of Concrete Operations

Children are limited by their lack of experience in life. They are constantly adding to their knowledge base of factual information, which they use to solve problems. Thinking concretely takes practice. Math and science problems, sorting stamps, building cities of Legos, and reading exercise the mind.

School-age children have difficulty with abstract reasoning, which involves using symbols that can be manipulated mentally to represent reality. For example, in algebra the symbol "*x*" represents different numbers in different problems. In literature, the grim reaper symbolizes death. Abstract thinking develops during adolescence.

Implications for Health Care Providers

Concrete thinkers conceptualize illness in terms of external cause and internal effect. Something outside, like cold water or germs, comes in contact with or enters the body, causing the body to malfunction, like a machine that is broken (Bibace and Walsh, 1981). Germs get into the nose and lungs and clog them up so that breathing is difficult. To fix it, reverse the sequence. Breathe warm air from a humidifier to push the germs out.

To concrete thinkers, a medical procedure is a sequence of predetermined steps. For example, they want to change a dressing the same way each time. Without the benefits of abstract thinking, they do not appreciate the principles of asepsis and wound healing that underlie the procedure, and have difficulty understanding that there may be more than 1 right way to do it. Using matrix classifications skills, older children with diabetes can learn to sort food groups and exchanges for their diets.

48 Intelligence

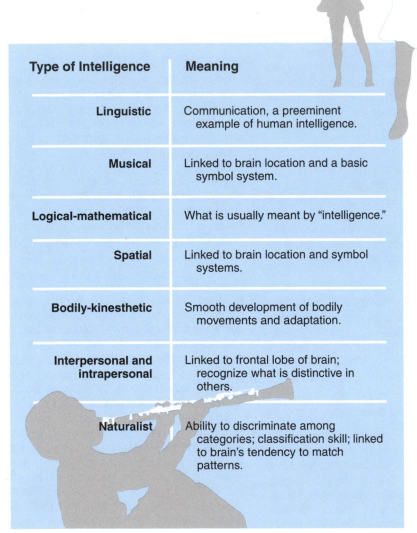

Type of Intelligence	Meaning
Linguistic	Communication, a preeminent example of human intelligence.
Musical	Linked to brain location and a basic symbol system.
Logical-mathematical	What is usually meant by "intelligence."
Spatial	Linked to brain location and symbol systems.
Bodily-kinesthetic	Smooth development of bodily movements and adaptation.
Interpersonal and intrapersonal	Linked to frontal lobe of brain; recognize what is distinctive in others.
Naturalist	Ability to discriminate among categories; classification skill; linked to brain's tendency to match patterns.

Recent Theories of Intelligence

Several recent theories have been proposed to explain intelligence and cognitive development. Two of these, Howard Gardner's theory of multiple intelligences and Robert Sternberg's triarchic model of intelligence, seem particularly significant.

The Theory of Multiple Intelligences

Howard Gardner's theory (1983, 1995, 1997) of *multiple intelligences* helps to explain the diverse abilities of individuals who are capable of penetrating mathematical vision but who are baffled by the most obvious musical symbols. To explain this phenomenon, Gardner identified 8 kinds of intelligence, any one of which may be outstanding in a particular individual (see **Table**).

1. *Linguistic intelligence.* Gardner's first category is linguistic intelligence—language. Studying damage to the language area of the brain, researchers have identified the core operations of any language (phonology, syntax, semantics, and pragmatics).
2. *Musical intelligence.* The early appearance of musical ability (in individuals such as Yehudi Menuhin) suggests a biological basis for musical intelligence. The right hemisphere of the brain seems particularly important for music, and musical notation clearly indicates a basic symbol system.
3. *Logical-mathematical intelligence.* Logical-mathematical intelligence is probably what most people think of as intelligence. Gardner used Piaget's ideas to trace the evolution of scientific thinking.
4. *Spatial intelligence.* Gardner believed that the abilities to perceive the visual world accurately, to manipulate initial perceptions, and to recreate aspects of visual experiences identify spatial intelligence. Spatial intelligence becomes obvious during middle childhood, as children produce advanced drawings, explain the relationships on a map, and excel at putting puzzles together.
5. *Bodily-kinesthetic intelligence.* Control of bodily motions and an ability to handle objects competently are indications of bodily-kinesthetic intelligence. It is clear that intelligence is a critical component of expert physical performance. During middle childhood, children's physical acts (throwing, catching, etc.) become highly coordinated. Some become so adept that even at this early age they are skilled athletes, dancers, and so on.
6, 7. *Interpersonal and intrapersonal intelligence.* These are the personal intelligences: Interpersonal intelligence builds on an ability to recognize what is distinctive in others, while intrapersonal intelligence enables people to understand their own feelings.
8. *Naturalist intelligence.* Gardner recently identified this eighth type of intelligence. It is the human ability to discriminate among living things as well as a sensitivity to the natural world.

Sternberg's Triarchic Model of Intelligence

Robert Sternberg (1988, 1990, 1994, 1996) designed a *triarchic model* of intelligence containing 3 major categories.

1. *The components of intelligence.* Sternberg's model contains 3 information-processing components:
   a. *Metacomponents*, which help individuals to plan, monitor, and evaluate problem-solving strategies (formulate certain steps to solve a problem)
   b. *Performance components*, which help individuals to execute the instructions of the metacomponents (go to the library for the needed information)
   c. *Knowledge-acquisition components*, which help individuals to learn how to solve problems in the first place (a particular way of studying—learning or cognitive style)

   These 3 components are highly interactive and generally act together. For example, let's assume you decide to write an outline for your developmental psychology course. The metacomponents help you to decide on the subjects to include, plan what to include, monitor the actual writing, and evaluate the final product. The performance components help you in the actual writing of the outline. You use the knowledge-acquisition components to do your research.
2. *Experience and intelligence.* Sternberg's second category refers to individual experiences, which improve the ability to deal with novel tasks and to use pertinent information to solve problems. On occasions when children must confront the unknown, their intelligence and problem-solving skills help them to face new challenges.
3. *The context of intelligence.* The context of intelligence is the ability to adapt to the various environments individuals move through in their culture. The major thrust of contextual intelligence is adaptation: Either individuals adjust to current circumstances, change these conditions to meet their needs, or move on to new circumstances.

Implications for Health Care Providers

The work of Gardner and Sternberg should encourage you to view teaching patients in a new light. Not everyone learns by reading about a disease, or by watching a demonstration of how to give an injection. Sternberg also reminds us that health teaching and learning are complex processes, not a rote exchange of information. It is important to understand how your clients learn so your teaching can become more effective.

49 Problem Solving

A

Two motorcyclists are 100 miles apart. At exactly the same moment, they begin to drive toward each other for a meeting. Just as they leave, a bird flies from the front of the first cyclist to the front of the second cyclist. When it reaches the second cyclist, it turns around and flies back to the first. The bird continues flying in this manner until the cyclists meet. The cyclists both travel at the rate of 50 miles per hour, while the bird maintains a constant speed of 75 miles per hour. How many miles will the bird have flown when the cyclists meet?

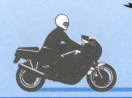 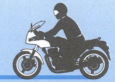

B

888 88 8 88 888 8

Group these numbers in such a way that when you
total the groups, they add up to the sum of 1,000.

88888888

8 8 88 8

888 88 88 888

During middle childhood, youngsters use their emerging cognitive accomplishments to solve the problems they face in their daily lives. A great deal is known about problem-solving strategies and this knowledge can be of great value to children. For example, simply reassuring them that there is nothing to be afraid of when they face a problem and urging them to look carefully for the facts that are given in a problem greatly improves their problem-solving abilities.

What Is a Problem?

Technically, a problem is a *significant discrepancy between the actual behavior and the desired behavior*. Children know a problem exists when they cannot get where they want to go; a gap stretches before them. To solve the problem, they must construct some way of bridging the gap.

The Kinds of Errors Children Make in Solving Problems

Children can improve their problem-solving ability if they become aware of the kinds of errors they make in attempting to solve problems, such as not attending to details or being uncertain about how to begin. Some of the more common traps that children—and adults—fall into include the following:

- **Failure to observe and use all the relevant facts of a problem.** Children must learn to constantly search the problem for all the information they can get (see **Part A**).
- **Failure to use systematic, step-by-step procedures.** Children often skip steps, ignore vital information, and leap to a faulty conclusion.
- **Failure to perceive vital relationships in the problem.** Children need to automatically search for patterns since that is how humans function.

Characteristics of Good Problem Solvers

Obviously some people are better at problem solving than others, owing to intelligence, experience, or education. However, it is possible to improve anyone's ability to solve problems, even children's.

- **Good problem solvers have a positive attitude toward problems,** believing they can solve them by careful, persistent analysis.
- **They are concerned with accuracy,** which is a wonderful attitude to foster in children, one that carries over to all aspects of their lives.
- **They learn to take a problem apart,** to break it down into its smallest, manageable parts, and then integrate the parts into a manageable whole that leads to a solution.

- **They learn not to guess and jump at answers,** a valuable tool to remember whenever they are challenged by a problem, in or out of school (see **Part B**).

These characteristics do not just appear. They require knowledge, work, and persistence. One way of helping children improve their problem-solving skills is by teaching them simple rules to follow, that is, a model of problem-solving behavior.

The DUPE Model

Many models have been proposed to help people solve a wide variety of problems. An easy acronym for children to remember is DUPE and its intent is to convey the message, *don't let yourself be deceived*. The meaning of each letter is described here.

D Is for Determine

Determine just exactly what the nature of the problem is. Too often, meaningless elements in the problem are deceptive; it is here that attention to detail is so important.

U Is for Understand

Understand the nature of the problem. Realizing that a particular problem exists is not enough; you must also comprehend the essence of the problem if your plan for solution is to be accurate.

P Is for Plan

Plan your solution. Now that you know that a problem exists and you understand its nature, you must select strategies that are appropriate for the problem. It is here that memory plays such an important role.

E Is for Evaluate

Evaluate your plan, which usually entails two phases. First you should examine the plan itself in an attempt to determine its suitability. Then you must decide how successful your solution was.

Implications for Health Care Providers

In your work with others, you typically find clients in a state of either physical or psychological stress. A major step in helping them toward recovery is to have clients believe that they have the capability of aiding themselves. Encourage them to see their present difficulty as a problem, and then help them to understand and use the strategies discussed in this chapter. The DUPE model is a particularly effective means of identifying a problem and devising steps for its solution.

50 Moral Development

Kohlberg's stages of moral development

Level I. Preconventional (about 4 10 years)

During these years children respond mainly to cultural control to avoid punishment and attain satisfaction. There are 2 stages:

Stage 1. Punishment and obedience. Children obey rules and orders to avoid punishment; there is no concern about moral rectitude.

Stage 2. Naive instrumental behaviorism. Children obey rules but only for pure self-interest; they are vaguely aware of fairness to others but obey rules for their own satisfaction. Kohlberg introduces the notion of reciprocity here: "You scratch my back, I'll scratch yours."

Level II. Conventional (about 10 13 years)

During these years children desire approval, both from individuals and from society. They not only conform, but also actively support society's standards. There are 2 stages:

Stage 3. Children seek the approval of others, the "good boy good girl" mentality. They begin to judge behavior by intention: "She meant to do well."

Stage 4. Law-and-order mentality. Children are concerned with authority and maintaining the social order. Correct behavior is "doing one's duty".

Level III. Postconventional (13 years and over)

If true morality (an internal moral code) is to develop, it appears during these years. The individual does not appeal to other people for moral decisions; these decisions are made by an "enlightened conscience". There are 2 stages:

Stage 5. An individual makes moral decisions legalistically or contractually; that is, the best values are those supported by the law because they have been accepted by the whole society. If there is a conflict between human need and the law, individuals should work to change the law.

Stage 6. An informed conscience decides what is right. People act, not from fear, approval, or law, but from their own internalized standards of right and wrong.

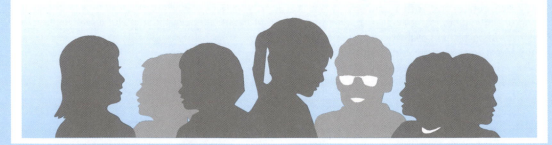

Moral development refers to the emergence in children of *universal* moral standards that lead to the condemnation of such behaviors as robbing, murdering, raping, and the like. *Conventional moral standards*, however, refers to the ideas that a particular group, religion, or culture believe in but cannot demand that everybody else agree with them. For example, in India violations of food taboos are regarded as seriously as crimes against a person. Those in Western cultures cannot accept this belief, but members of both cultures agree in condemning murder. Culture, with its powerful influence on conventional moral standards, is a recurrent theme in any analysis of moral development.

As we begin our analysis of children's moral progress, keep in mind that moral behavior is a complex mixture of *cognition* (thinking about what to do), *emotion* (feelings about what to do or what was done), and *behavior* (what is actually done).

The Pattern of Moral Growth

Young children (birth to about 2 or 3 years) begin to learn about right and wrong from their parents and during these early years, modeling is especially effective. Lacking cognitive sophistication, young children who have a good relationship with their parents usually are impressed by what they see their parents doing.

The next phase (about 2–6 years) reflects children's growing cognitive maturity and their developing ability to decide what is right or wrong.

As children move into middle childhood (about 6–12 years), they interact with their siblings in their family lives, with their schoolmates in classroom experiences, and with their friends in games and other social activities. Here they again encounter the reality of rules, rules not established by parental edict. Consequently, they learn about making and following regulations as well as deriving insights into the children who don't.

Can Children Be Moral Philosophers?

Lawrence Kohlberg believed children can be moral. Fascinated with the study of children's moral development during his doctoral work at the University of Chicago, especially Piaget's work, Kohlberg developed his ideas by presenting children with a series of moral dilemmas and then asking them *what* they would do and *why* they would do it. The dilemmas were real or imaginary conflicts that forced children to make decisions based on their moral reasoning.

Kohlberg found that children begin to think about moral issues at about the age of 4 years as they pass through 3 levels of moral development. Each of these levels contains 2 stages; thus there are 3 levels and 6 stages of moral development. Take a few moments and study the levels and stages in the **Table** (Kohlberg, 1966).

Remember, however, even children who make it to the third level as adults may not always act in a moral manner. Knowing the right answer to a moral dilemma does not guarantee moral behavior, which is why we distinguished among knowing, feeling, and behaving earlier in the chapter. A person may be brilliant, but also morally destitute.

Gender and Moral Development

Gilligan (1977, 1982, 1988) questioned the validity of Kohlberg's theory for women. She believed that Kohlberg's theory stressed the moral qualities of masculinity (autonomous thinking, clear decision making, and responsible action) and ignored those associated with femininity. For example, the characteristics that define the traditional "good woman" (gentleness, tact, concern for others, display of feelings) all contribute to a different concept of morality.

Gilligan (1988, p. 7) argued strongly that different images of self lead to different interpretations of moral behavior. Girls, raised with the belief that attachment is desirable, fuse the experience of attachment (see Chapter 29) with the process of identity formation.

Consequently, since women's moral decisions are based on an *ethic of caring* rather than a *morality of justice*, Gilligan argued for a different interpretation of moral development for women. For males, *separation from mothers* is essential to the development of masculinity, whereas for females, femininity is defined by *attachment to mothers*. Male gender identity is threatened by attachment, whereas female gender identity is threatened by separation. Women define themselves through a context of human relationships and judge themselves by their ability to care (Gilligan, 1982, p. 17).

Implications for Health Care Providers

Lying, stealing, and cheating are common temptations for all children and should not be tolerated. In some cases, however, they may indicate serious behavioral disturbances. Parents may express concerns during a routine visit, or you may hear children complain about a peer. Moral behavior is learned in a number of ways, but you do your part when you model honesty, fairness, and taking responsibility for your behavior.

Typical language accomplishments: 6–10 years

Age (yr)	Language Accomplishments
6	Has vocabulary of several thousand words; understands complex sentences; uses language as a tool; possesses some reading ability
	Is able to print several sentences; begins to tell time; losing tendency to reverse letters (*b*, *d*)
	Can write as well as print; understands that words may have more than 1 meaning (ball)
	Describes objects in detail; writes well; uses sentence content to determine word meaning
12	Describes situations by cause and effect; writes fairly lengthy essays; likes mystery and science stories; masters dictionary skills; good sense of grammar

By middle childhood, most children have acquired the critical components of their language and find themselves engulfed in a verbal world. During middle childhood, both vocabulary and structural knowledge continue to expand. By the end of the period, children are similar to adults in their language usage. Children who experience language problems are at a serious disadvantage with their peers, at school, and in their overall relationships with others.

The Language Expert

During middle childhood children communicate with others more effectively and realize that language is a powerful tool they can use to manipulate their world. Increasing visual discrimination is apparent in the accurate description of events and the elimination of letter reversals (e.g., *b* for *d*). Growth in cognitive ability is seen in the detection of cause and effect, and the appeal of science and mystery stories.

As their vocabulary continues to grow, children begin to demonstrate divergent and convergent language abilities. *Divergent semantic production* is seen in the wide variety of words, phrases, and sentences they use when discussing a topic, thus bringing originality, flexibility, and creativity to their language. *Convergent semantic production* is seen when children use the right word in response to a specific, restricted question such as, What is the opposite of hot (Owens, 1996)?

Bilingual Education

Today there are over 30 million Americans for whom English is not their primary language and of them about 6 million have *limited English proficiency* (LEP). About 10 million children of school age are not fluent in English (Reagan, 1997). Of those who have some knowledge of English, many use variations that render their oral language almost unintelligible. Consequently, no discussion of language development is complete without mentioning the efforts underway to help LEP children.

Many children who do not speak the language of their school are taught by teachers who have no special proficiency or training in working with these children. Unfortunately, many children will achieve below their potential and drop out of school. In an effort to combat this problem, the *Bilingual Education Act of 1988* stipulated that students with LEP receive *bilingual education* until they can use English to succeed in school.

Bilingual Children

The better that children speak both languages, the better their level of cognitive attainment is. The native language does not interfere with the second language since the phonemic categories of the first language serve as a basis for learning the second language. Many adjustments are made in learning the second language (Hakuta and McLaughlin, 1996).

Since the acquisition of languages is a natural part of the cognitive system, both first- and second-language acquisition seems to be guided by similar principles. In fact, the rate of acquisition of the second language seems to be related to the level of proficiency of the first. With these ideas in mind, programs have been devised to help these children.

Bilingual Education Programs

Two different techniques for aiding LEP students are apparent:

- The *English as a Second Language* (ESL) program usually has students removed from the class and given special English instruction.
- With the *bilingual* technique, students are taught partly in English and partly in their native language. The objective is to help students learn English by subject matter instruction in their own language and also in English.

Bilingual education programs can be divided into 2 categories. First, some programs (often called "transitional" programs) encourage the rapid development of English so that students switch as soon as possible to an all-English program. The second type of program (sometimes referred to as "maintenance" programs) permits LEP students to remain in the program even after they have become proficient in English. The rationale for such programs is that students can use both languages to develop mature skills and to become fully bilingual.

Since the use of 2 languages in classroom instruction actually is bilingual education, several important questions arise:

- What acceptable level of English signals the end of a student's participation?
- What subjects should be taught in each language?
- How can each language be used most effectively? (That is, how much of each language is to be used to help a student's progress with school subjects?)
- Should English be gradually phased in, or should students be totally immersed in the second language (which, for most of the students we are discussing, would be English)?

Implications for Health Care Providers

In your work, you will occasionally meet children of this age with speech or language difficulties. Be alert for any articulation disorders, problems with the flow of speech, or speech usage that differs from that of typical children. If one of your clients has some type of language difficulty, reinforce his or her verbal and nonverbal attempts at communication as carefully as possible. You should be a model of clear and correct language usage.

52 Peers and Social Development

A Key terms

Social cognition: ability to read a social situation.

Egocentric: sees social situations mostly from one's own point of view but can empathize.

Unilateral: when the perspective on a relationship is one-way; " I know you have thoughts and feelings, but mine count more."

Second-person perspective: the ability to see things from another person's social and emotional point of view; reciprocity.

Third-person perspective: the ability to step back and observe one's self in a situation involving others; mutuality.

B Stages of social-emotional development

Age 3–6	
A friend ...	is who I played with today; won't break my toys.
Perspective	Egocentric: "world is my oyster"; reads actions, not intentions.
Conflict	Is intrusive; impulse hitting; running away.
Feelings	Feelings are outside; smile means happy; feelings associated with events.
Age 5–9	
A friend ...	likes the same things as me; "Let's do this."
Perspective	Unilateral: "I win"; I know you have feelings, intents.
Conflict	You vs me; do this or else; "Do what I say or I'll tell the teacher."
Feelings	I can hide feelings inside, so can you; events cause feelings.
Age 7–12	
A friend ...	who likes me and has the same experiences as me; won't leave me out; keeps secrets.
Perspective	Reciprocal, 2nd-person perspective; I put myself in your shoes, you can put yourself in mine.
Conflict	Between me and you, I'll get you to see it my way; guilt tripping; persuasion.
Feelings	I have more than one feeling about an event; I can pretend to feel angry in order to fool you.
Age 8–15	
A friend ...	works to keep our friendship going; knows who I am.
Perspective	Mutual, 3rd-person perspective: I see our friendship as part of a whole.
Conflict	Between us, work it out so solution benefits both of us.
Feelings	Express multiple conflicting feelings; introspective; not sure how I feel.

While the attitude of younger children is "the world is my oyster," for school-age children, "the world is other kids" (Greenspan, 1993). Peers are central to children's development. Whereas their relationships with adults and with children younger and older than themselves are vertical in nature, and reflect a hierarchy of experience and authority, their relationships with peers are more horizontal (Hartup, 1983). Peers may not be equal in ability or expertise or the same age. They are of roughly equal status in the give-and-take of a relationship, the context for development of social and moral reasoning.

Concept of Friendship and Perspective Taking

How children think about themselves and friendships is related to cognitive development, and to the ability to take someone else's point of view (Selman and Schultz, 1991) (see **Part A** and **Part B**).

Children ages 3–6 are aware that other people have feelings but they focus on what other people do and not their subjective experiences or intentions. Friendships are momentary physical interactions. Friends are people they played with this morning. Trust means their friend won't break their toys. Young children ascribe their own feelings to others. When shopping for a present for someone else, children will buy something they themselves want.

During the early school years, friendships are less egocentric and more unilateral. Children are aware of subjective experiences in others, but their own interests predominate. Friends like the things "I" like to do. "He didn't play fair" really means "He didn't do what I wanted." Teasing is an obnoxious type of verbal dominance behavior, and if left unchecked, turns into harassment.

By age 10, the development of a second-person perspective allows children to put themselves in other people's shoes and experience things from their point of view. They expect that friends will do the same for them. Children realize that if they can hide feelings and thoughts, so can others; social appearances can be deceiving. Friendships expand beyond sharing activities to sharing subjective experiences. Trust means they won't hurt their friend's feelings, that they understand the desire to be liked and accepted. Hurting people's feelings is understood to be intentional. Being excluded is painful.

Recognizing different perspectives means concrete thinkers can compare themselves with others. No longer is everybody the fastest runner; there can be only one. Older school-age children who reflect on their own abilities and feelings relative to others become very self-conscious. They are also very effective teachers for younger children and less-able peers because they are so attuned to the other's experience.

Social Cognition

Social cognition is the ability to read a social situation, and decide how to act accordingly. Whereas social cognition reflects underlying levels of cognitive development, social skills develop with experience, practice, and guidance. How well or poorly children learn these skills determines their popularity and classroom performance, and affects self-concept.

Because preschool children focus on what is happening right now, they resolve conflict by trying to alter circumstances. They impulsively act out, grab toys or impulsively withdraw, run away, or shut down emotionally. The consequences tell children that hitting is socially unacceptable, and running away solves nothing (Selman and Schultz, 1991).

In the early school years, conflict is experienced as unilateral dominance, that is, "me against you" and "you started it!" The outcomes of unilateral social strategies are designed to favor only 1 of us—me. They include verbal commands and threats, or acting victimized, and appealing to powerful others (like teachers) to intervene (Selman and Schultz, 1991).

An appreciation for the second-person perspective during the later school years opens the door to new social skills. If I can see things from your point of view, I can persuade you to see them from mine. I might use my inadequacy as a tool to make you feel guilty. I could do it your way, and next time you'll do it my way. Or let's figure out a way to make it work for everybody (Selman and Schultz, 1991). Influence, persuasion, and negotiation are sophisticated strategies that sustain friendships and activities among peers.

The Games Children Play

The school-age years are the period of "playground politics" because children learn to negotiate the complex social structure of the peer group (Greenspan, 1993). Alliances shift. The rough and tumble play and physical aggression of early childhood give way to competitive games of mental and physical skill. School-age children are inflexible about the rules of competition because rules are a civilized way of resolving conflict and keeping aggressive tendencies in check. Competition can foster the development of social, mental, and physical skills through friendly rivalry, but when the only goal is to win, competition fosters dominance behavior. Children need cooperative and competence-building activities. Hobbies, Girl and Boy Scout troops, and chores around the house promote cooperation, problem solving, and self-confidence.

A Some developmental tasks of middle childhood

Physical	Learning the physical skills necessary for games
Cognitive	Building a healthy self-concept Learning an appropriate sex role Developing the fundamental skills Ñ reading, writing, arithmetic Developing concepts for everyday living
Social	Learning to get along with others Learning an appropriate sex role Developing acceptable attitudes toward society
Personal-Emotional	Building a healthy self-concept Developing attitudes and values Achieving independence

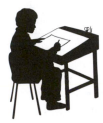

B National educational goals

- By the year 2000, all children in America will start school ready to learn.
- By the year 2000, the high school graduation rate will increase to at least 90%.
- By the year 2000, all children will leave grades 4, 8, and 12 having demonstrated competency over challenging subject matter.
- By the year 2000, U.S. students will be first in the world in mathematics and science achievement.
- By the year 2000, every adult American will be literate and will possess the knowledge and skills to compete in a global economy and exercise the rights and responsibilities of citizenship.
- By the year 2000, every school in America will be free of drugs, violence, and the unauthorized presence of firearms and alcohol and will offer a disciplined environment conducive to learning.
- By the year 2000, the nation's teaching force will have access to programs for the continued improvement of their professional skills.
- By the year 2000, every school will promote partnerships that will increase parental involvement and participation.

Schooling is important at any time in a child's life, but developmentally appropriate instruction and materials are crucial during middle childhood. We know that children's talents—abilities in science or mathematics, artistic talent, musical capability, and athletic skill—become apparent between ages 6 and 11. **Part A** lists developmental tasks of middle childhood (note that several of these tasks cross domains).

Much is expected of schools today and, in spite of dramatic headlines, much has been accomplished (see **Part B**). But all the pro and con arguments about school, come down to one basic: Do schools make a difference?

Schools *Do* Make A Difference

Schools make a profound difference in children's lives. During the past 20–25 years, a substantial body of literature has sharply defined the characteristics marking an effective school. With colleagues, Michael Rutter (1979), an internationally respected researcher of children's issues, in a massive and meticulously conducted study of school effectiveness, found startling differences between schools. The data led to several conclusions:

- Children were more likely to show good behavior and good scholastic achievement when they attended some schools but not others.
- Differences between the schools were not due to the size or age of the buildings, or the space available.
- Differences between the schools were due to a school's emphasis on academic success, teacher expectations of student success, time-on-task, skillful use of rewards and punishment, teachers who provided a comfortable and warm classroom environment, and teachers who insisted on student responsibility for their behavior.

These criteria graphically demonstrate that *good instructional leadership* is critical, which means that principals, teachers, students, and parents agree on goals, methods, and content. Home-school cooperation supports good leadership, which in turn produces an *orderly environment* that fosters desirable discipline, academic success, and personal fulfillment. When teachers sense the support of parents and administrators, they intuitively respond in a manner that promotes student achievement and adjustment, encourages collegiality among teachers, and produces a warm, yet exciting atmosphere.

What We Know about Our Schools

President John Kennedy once said that life is unfair. He was right—unfortunately, defective schools do exist. When visiting less-effective schools, an observer is immediately struck by the lack of communication among all the leading players. Everyone and everything seem compartmentalized. Students lack commitment to the school itself or its teachers, teachers lack any degree of collegiality, issues are not discussed, and decisions are rendered from above. Parental involvement is actively discouraged.

The outstanding features that characterize high-achieving schools are as follows:

- A moderately authoritarian principal who works well with parents. The school's leader should have well-defined educational objectives and the motivation, inclination, and skill to achieve them.
- A principal who does not fear to be different in order to help students achieve to the best of their ability. A creative and realistic leader can help children to explore new and exciting topics, which can only heighten students' positive feelings toward school.
- A community that agrees with the school about high achievement as the top-priority objective. Principals and teachers should be sensitive to the need for jointly (parents, teachers, administrators) formulated school goals since cooperation between home and school can only further children's achievement and adjustment.
- An educational environment that has high expectations for student achievement. The critical role that expectations play in children's achievement has been a consistent finding of the research. When children know that much is expected of them, they respond to the challenge as well as their ability permits.
- Clearly stated rules and regulations that help students realize their goals. Well-run schools have a few basic rules that children know, understand, and follow. These serve as a guide to acceptable school behavior.
- Teachers, principals, and parents who are willing to fight for the policies and programs that lead to high achievement.

Implications for Health Care Providers

Schools and health care have long functioned in separate realms. The link between the 2 has typically been the school nurse, whose duties have been restricted to public health initiatives (immunization schedules, emergency needs of individual students). Since good health is linked to school success, schools should integrate student health issues with academic initiatives.

Common Characteristics of Creativity

Tolerant of ambiguity	Insightful	Intuitive
Flexible	Visual ability	Self-critical
Original	Fluent	Risk taking
Intelligent	Sensitive	Knowledgeable
Independent	Imaginative	Analytical
Able to synthesize	Connected	Curious
Persistent	Resilient	Focused

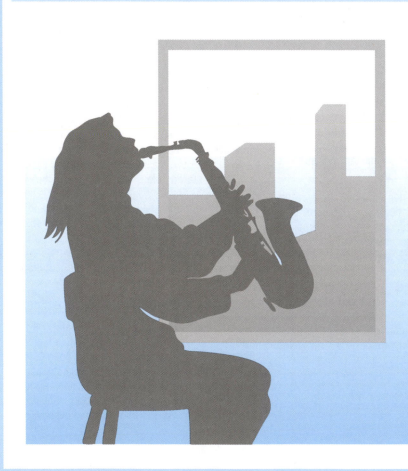

The essential ingredients of creativity: include an inquiring mind, a supportive environment, a willingness to look at problems from a different perspective, determination that could not be extinguished, and an acceptance of the risks accompanying novel ventures. But it isn't only academic or scientific fields that thirst for creative ideas; the way we relate to each other demands creativity too. The strains of modern living frequently necessitate a new way of looking at relationships, which involves just as much creativity as the work Edison was engaged in. Can children, growing up in a modern society, retain that spark of creativity that adds a dynamic dimension to their lives?

Characteristics of Creative Children

Most creative people exhibit several characteristics:

- **Creative people learn the strategies needed to solve the problems they inevitably encounter.**
- **Creative people don't quit when the going gets tough; they persevere.**
- **Creative people are sensitive to problems.**
- ***Creative people are more fluent than most other people.*** (They generate a large number of ideas, which is called "ideational fluency.")
- **Creative people propose novel ideas that are also useful.**
- **Creative people demonstrate considerable flexibility of mind.**
- **Creative people reorganize the elements.**

The **Table** summarizes the more common characteristics of creativity.

The Creative Process

Three elements are particularly important for understanding the creative process: *knowledge, visualization*, and the *thinking process* itself.

Knowledge

Information is one of the critical necessities of the creative process. Some children are usually more interested in one subject than others. For example, some children are drawn almost immediately to physical activities in which they show early grace, skill, and coordination. Other children turn almost intuitively to artistry and demonstrate early talent. Still others are highly verbal almost from the time they begin to talk. Consequently, children need to acquire vital fundamental knowledge.

Visualization

Three kinds of visual thinking cut to the heart of the creative process (McKim, 1972):

1. *Perceptual imagery.* Children do not respond to their surroundings on a one-to-one basis. For example, when someone asks you what time it is, do you carefully scrutinize all of the minute markings and the second hand on your watch? No, your familiarity with telling time leads you immediately to the important section where the hands and numbers are. Children do exactly the same thing; that is, they try to form meaningful patterns to help them understand everything going on around them.

2. *Mental imagery.* The information children obtain from their perceptual imagery is stored in the form of a representation. The word *car* is a representation; it *represents* a certain idea (something with wheels, that moves, etc.). Given the tremendous flexibility children have with language, the representation of this object could be stored in many other forms: *auto, automobile,* or *wheels.* For each form, however, the information represented remains the same.

3. *Graphic imagery.* Sometimes merely seeing the pieces of a puzzle, or visualizing how words or symbols connect to each other, or even sketching the physical location of people and seeing how they relate to each other will change a pattern and put individuals on the track to solve whatever problem they are dealing with.

Implications for Health Care Providers

AIDS research? Causes of cancer? Urban renewal? Diplomatic breakthroughs? Just think of what is needed to solve these problems: enormous knowledge stored in the researcher's memory; the ability to identify crucial relationships in the information; the availability of strategies to attack the problem; a talent for visualizing patterns in a vast array of data; and finally, the skill to recombine elements, that is, move A to M, M to Z, and Z to A. If children's creativity is encouraged early in their lives, they will learn to apply creative thinking to the problems they face, helping them to enjoy richer, more meaningful lives.

55 Resilience in Childhood

A Risk and protective factors in disadvantaged children

Risk Factors	Protective Factors
Child	**Child**
Male	Female
Irritable, hyperactive	Easy-going personality
Poor self-control	Good self-control
Learning impairment	Good cognitive skills
Poor social skills	Good social skills
Difficulty making friends	Has friends
Family	**Family**
Family discord/divorce	Cohesive family
Criminal activity in father	Network of friends
Mental illness in mother	Competent mother
Overcrowded living space	Religious affiliation
>4 children, spaced <2 yr apart	<4 children, spaced >2 yr apart
Community	**Community**
Poor school environment	School/community programs
No positive adult role models	Adult guidance

B Risk and protective factors in adaptation to chronic illness

Risk Factors: Disease/Disability	Resistance Factors
Functional dependence	Child: social competence, problem-solving
Involvement of brain	skills, stress appraisal and coping
Impaired cognitive functioning	Social: cohesive family, support for mother,
Poor bowel/bladder control	social network,
Visible, especially the face	practical resources (money, insurance)
Chronicity, daily hassles	child has friends, activities

We are interested in resilience for 2 reasons. First, developmentalists believe there are sensitive periods for attaining certain milestones, for example, attachment. When circumstances interfere with development, how far off the normal developmental path can children stray before the likelihood of recovery is lost? Second, it is important to learn what factors contribute to resilience among children subject to chronic stress from poverty, abuse, or illness.

Deprivation and Trauma: How Far off the Path?

We learn about the effects of deprivation on development by studying children who have been subject to it and then rescued. The story of Genie, a girl in California, is well known. She was tied up alone in a locked room by her father between ages 2 and 13. Food was left but no one spoke to her. When rescued, she could not walk, was not toilet trained, made no sounds, and displayed no emotion. With care, her health recovered, and she became responsive to selected people. She never developed normal language, and has lasting cognitive deficits.

In Czechoslovakia, twin boys were locked away together as toddlers. Rescued at age 6, they could barely talk and lagged cognitively. Unlike Genie, they displayed fear and wariness. Placed in a home for younger children with whom they could more easily interact, they were adopted and recovered developmentally by age 14 (Koluchova, 1976).

In Lebanon, babies were abandoned in orphanages and were left to languish in cribs. Those adopted before age 2 recovered. Those adopted at age 4 fared slightly less well. Those subjected to deprivation throughout childhood were functionally retarded by adolescence (Dennis, 1973).

These cases indicate that the sensitive period for attachment can be extended to age 4 and language development to age 6 if followed by high-quality nurturing. They also illustrate the importance of a biopsychosocial model for understanding development. The deprived Lebanese orphans strayed further from the normal developmental path than did the Koluchova twins. The twins were developing normally prior to their ordeal, they were confined together and not socially isolated, and received optimal care afterward. The orphans were subject to prolonged deprivation.

Chronic Stress: Risk and Protective Factors

Studies of children subjected to chronic adversity have identified what factors increase the risk of poor developmental outcome and what factors protect against the same risk (see **Part A**). For example, children at greatest risk for abuse are those with health problems, especially premature infants; are under age 3; have irritable, defiant, or hyperactive personalities; and come from homes chronically stressed by poverty. Girls suffer more sexual abuse than boys. Estimates are that 2 million children a year are seriously abused in the United States.

The Isle of Wight studies in England identified 4 risk factors that contribute to delinquency, school failure, and mental health problems: (1) serious family discord; (2) parental deviance (criminal activity, mental illness); (3) low socioeconomic status, overcrowded living conditions; and (4) poor school environment (Rutter et al., 1975). Negative effects are not additive but multiplicative, that is, having 2 factors increases the risk 400%, not 200%. Boys are at greater risk than girls.

In the longitudinal study of the disadvantaged children on the island of Kauai in Hawaii, 30% have prospered better than expected. Children who are resilient have good cognitive and social skills, and easy-going personalities that attract adults and peers, who in turn provide guidance and friendship. Families are cohesive, with a multigenerational network of family members and friends who help care for children. The network provides structure, rules, and expectations (e.g., household chores, caring for siblings, doing homework, etc.). Though poorly educated, mothers of resilient children often work outside the home, providing children with competent role models. Resilient children come from communities in which there are adult-run church and school programs, and health clinics (Werner and Smith, 1992).

Families of children with chronic illness and disability have similar risk and protective factors (see **Part B**). Poor developmental outcome is linked to unresolved family discord, lack of structure and organization, lower socioeconomic class, and functional dependence on parents by the child for routine care, such as feeding. Contrary to popular belief, severity of illness or disability alone is not a factor.

Factors that protect children with health problems include families that are cohesive and organized, and that promote autonomy. Families are connected to the community through work. The better educated the mother, the better off the child. Educated mothers are adept at finding the resources medically ill children need, and the family is of a higher socioeconomic class (Kronenberger and Thompson, 1990).

Theories of Resilience

Resilience should not be confused with being "hardy" or "invulnerable." It is not a character trait, but a dynamic process arising from interactions between children and the events and people in their lives. The key characteristic of resilience in children is connectedness—to family, friends, and other adults who can provide guidance, hope, and stability. Serendipity also plays a role. In some family circumstances, being the oldest child is a protective factor; in others, it carries risk.

Resilience does not imply that there are no harmful effects from adversity. In the face of adversity, resilient children and families are better able to reorganize, and to stay on the developmental path.

56 Exceptional Children

A Triangle of developmental disabilities

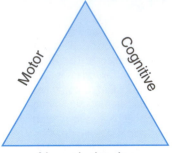

Motor

Cognitive

Neurobehavior

B

Common Disabilities	Common Illnesses	Laws to Know
Autism	Asthma (4.3%)	1973: Section 504 of the
Blind, vision disorders	Cancer	Rehabilitation Act
Deaf, hearing impairments	Cystic fibrosis	1975: PL 142-92 IDEA
Cerebral palsy	Diabetes	1990: ADA
Down syndrome	Hemophilia	1997: Reauthorization of IDEA
Mental retardation	Juvenile rheumatoid arthritis	Medicaid laws (by state)
Spina bifida	Sickle-cell anemia	Social Security (by state)

C Three-ring concept of giftedness

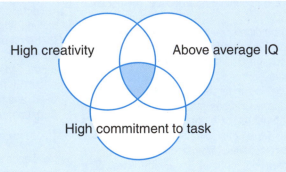

High creativity

Above average IQ

High commitment to task

D Key terms

Disability (ADA): physical or mental impairment that limits 1 or more major life activities, such as breathing, walking, seeing, hearing, and so on.

Other health impaired (IDEA): limited strength, vitality or alertness due to chronic or acute health problems, which adversely affect a child's educational performance.

Inclusion: philosophy that all children should be educated together, live in the same communities, and play together regardless of disability or health status.

Human development unfolds sequentially, and development in 1 area is tied to development in other areas. Play behavior shows an integration of language, visuomotor, and problem-solving skills. Not all children follow the typical developmental path. Four groups are exceptions.

According to the Social Securities Act of 1985, "children with special health care needs" account for 3 overlapping groups: developmental disabilities, mental retardation, and learning disabilities; chronic illness, such as diabetes and asthma; and emotional/behavioral difficulties, including attention deficit disorder (ADD). The fourth group of exceptional children are gifted in intellectual, artistic, or athletic abilities.

Developmental Disabilities, Mental Retardation, and Learning Disabilities

Developmental disabilities represent alterations in the typical developmental sequence in 1 or more of 3 areas: motor, cognitive, and neurobehavior (see **Part A**). *Motor* includes gross-motor, fine-motor, and visuomotor coordination. *Cognitive* includes central processing, problem solving, and language. *Neurobehavior* refers to self-help, self-regulatory, and social skills. These developmental disabilities are characterized by delay, dissociation, and/or deviation from the norm (Capute and Accardo, 1996).

A *developmental delay* is a significant lag in meeting milestones; for example, motor delays may indicate cerebral palsy. *Dissociation* is a difference between the rate of development in 2 aspects of 1 area, for example, between expressive and receptive language in children who are deaf. When the sequence of development in 1 or more areas deviates sufficiently from the norm, the overall pattern that emerges over time represents a different developmental path. In children with autism, development of language, social, and problem-solving skills is so skewed that the pattern of play behavior and peer interactions that emerges is very different.

Mental retardation is characterized by "subaverage intellectual functioning" along with limitations in 2 or more adaptive skills (e.g., academics, communication, ability to live on one's own, social skills, leisure, and work.) Mental retardation is 1 type, and is a distinctive feature of Fragile X, Down, and fetal alcohol syndromes. The definition reflects a new approach that broadens the previous emphasis on IQ scores to include abilities and adaptive skills.

Learning disabilities are characterized by a discrepancy between ability as measured on intelligence tests and actual achievement. The most common learning disabilities involve language function and metacognitive abilities, such as memory and problem solving. It is estimated that 3%–15% of school children have a learning disability (Parker and Zuckerman, 1995).

Chronic Medical Illness and Chronic Health Conditions

Chronic health conditions are biologically based, involve organ systems, and last for at least 3–12 months. They compromise day-to-day functioning; and/or require special diets, medications, or assistive devices; and/or require more health care than is routine. As many as 30% of people under age 21 have one of a wide range of chronic health conditions, which include disabilities and chronic illness (see **Part B**); prevalence is highest among the rural poor. About 6%–15% of youth have a chronic illness, which includes diabetes, cancer, hemophilia, and so on. Asthma affects 4% of American children.

Behavioral/Emotional Difficulties

Self-regulation in response to demands from people, settings, and events is key to adaptive behavior. While many children occasionally have difficulties, about 9% of children have serious conduct disorders, and 4%–6% have attention deficit hyperactivity disorder (ADHD). Posttraumatic stress disorder (PTSD) is found in children who have been abused. Prevalence of behavior and attention disorders is higher in boys and in lower socioeconomic groups. Treatment of ADHD is controversial. It is easier to medicate a child with Ritalin (methylphenidate) than to change the classroom environment (Parker and Zuckerman, 1995).

About 2% of children and 5% of adolescents are clinically depressed. Depression in youth is underdiagnosed by health professionals, who minimize the symptoms as a passing phase or a natural response to a stressful event. Untreated, it leads to social withdrawal, school failure, self-destructive behavior, and suicide.

Being Gifted

The definition of *gifted* has 3 intersecting parts (see **Part C**): above-average IQ, high levels of creativity, and high levels of commitment to a task. Giftedness is manifested in academics, creative thinking, leadership, visual/performing arts, and psychomotor abilities. About 5% of children can be considered gifted, which should not be confused with precociousness. Being gifted does not guarantee later success. Motivation, opportunity, and diligence play a role (Parker and Zuckerman, 1995).

Social Policy Issues

The emphasis must be on the child first and the condition second. The accepted reference is to "children with mental retardation" and not "retarded children." Children are not "cancer victims" nor do they "suffer" from spina bifida. Advocates are also responsible for a wide range of reform efforts.

The Individuals with Disabilities Education Act of 1975 (IDEA; reauthorized by Congress in 1997) allows children with disabilities to be educated in local schools rather than warehoused in institutions. It includes a category of disability called "other health impaired," which addresses children with chronic illness. The Americans with Disabilities Act of 1990 (ADA) makes it illegal to discriminate against people with disabilities, especially in the workplace and in school (see **Part D**).

Directions: For each of the following questions, choose the **one best** answer.

1. By what age can children typically ride a 2-wheel bicycle?

(A) 5 years

(B) 7 years

(C) 9 years

(D) 11 years

2. Malnourished American children tend to be obese, not thin, because

(A) they consume a lot of junk food.

(B) they watch too much TV.

(C) they eat too many packaged foods.

(D) of all of the above.

3. What did Piaget mean by "concrete operations"?

(A) Children's thinking is perceptually bound.

(B) Causal reasoning is based on association.

(C) Children's thinking is very matter of fact.

(D) Children can do mentally what had to be done physically before.

4. Boys of about ages 9–10 love to collect and sort baseball cards. What characteristic of concrete thought contributes to this activity?

(A) Hierarchical classification skills

(B) Matrix classification skills

(C) Abstract thinking

(D) Set identity

5. Sternberg's theory is based on

(A) context.

(B) gender.

(C) age.

(D) biology.

6. Gardner's theory of intelligence includes _____ types of equal intelligence.

(A) 2

(B) 4

(C) 6

(D) 8

7. A well-known model of problem solving is

(A) HOME.

(B) DUPE.

(C) NATO.

(D) SAC.

8. Everyone should attempt to internally represent solutions to problems.

(A) True

(B) False

(C) Uncertain

9. Kohlberg used a method called

(A) cognitive structuring.

(B) contextual determinism.

(C) moral dilemmas.

(D) contingencies of reinforcement.

10. Gilligan believed that Kohlberg's work was too _____ oriented.

(A) age

(B) culture

(C) neutral

(D) male

11. LEP refers to those students whose primary language is not

(A) English.

(B) Spanish.

(C) French.

(D) Vietnamese.

12. To work with LEP students, many school systems are trying to decide between ESL programs and

(A) separate systems.

(B) bilingual education.

(C) native-born instructors.

(D) curricular insertion.

13. By about what age do children develop reciprocity in their friendships?

(A) 6 years

(B) 8 years

(C) 10 years

(D) 12 years

14. Which of the following statements best describes children's games during middle childhood?

(A) Children are inflexible about the rules of competition.

(B) Rules help to keep aggression in check.

(C) Competition can foster social, mental, and physical development.

(D) All of the above are correct.

15. Good schools are characterized by their emphasis on

(A) building conditions.

(B) recreational facilities.

(C) amount of materials.

(D) academic success.

16. The author of an influential study of school effectiveness was

(A) Rutter.

(B) Piaget.

(C) Bruner.

(D) Skinner.

17. Creativity is also known as

(A) critical thinking.

(B) convergent thinking.

(C) divergent thinking.

(D) vertical thinking.

18. Among the characteristics of creativity are visualization, thinking processes, and

(A) knowledge.

(B) contingency.

(C) laterality.

(D) symmetry.

19. What is the sensitive period for the development of language?

(A) Up to 2 years old

(B) Up to 4 years old

(C) Up to 6 years old

(D) Up to 8 years old

20. What triad of factors contributes to resilience in children at risk?

(A) Family discord, low socioeconomic status, poor school environment

(B) Cohesive family, easy-going personality, competent adults in community

(C) Mothers who work, absent fathers, good social skills

(D) Being in foster care, concerned case worker, visits with mother

21. Developmental disabilities represent alterations in the typical developmental sequence of which 3 areas?

(A) Fine motor, gross motor, intelligence

(B) Problem solving, language, motor coordination

(C) Motor, cognitive, neurobehavior

(D) Neurobehavior, intelligence, gross motor

22. Which of the following describes children who are gifted?

(A) Above-average IQ

(B) High levels of creativity

(C) High levels of commitment to a task

(D) All of the above

PART V: ANSWERS AND EXPLANATIONS

1. The answer is B.

The organization of the CNS is like that in adults, contributing to better physical coordination. There is an increase in muscle mass relative to body weight. Body proportions change during the school years. Children have a lower center of gravity. There is an increase in leg length, decrease in head size, and decrease in waist size relative to height. These changes all contribute to physical agility, so that riding a bike, kicking a soccer ball, or hiking a mountain trail is easier and more coordinated.

2. The answer is D.

Malnourished American children tend to be obese, not thin, because they consume too much fat and sugar, mostly in junk foods. Their families use more high-fat, low-cost packaged foods, like macaroni and cheese, and eat fewer fresh fruits and vegetables. Also, the average child who watches 4 hours of television a day is not playing outside, expending energy, strengthening muscles and bones, and increasing aerobic capacity.

3. The answer is D.

In school-age children, concrete operational thinking consists of mental operations that allow children to do mentally what had to be experienced physically before. Actions can be played out in their minds, giving them more flexibility for solving problems than during the preschool years. Concrete thought is characterized by decreasing centration, reversibility of a mental sequence, set identity, conservation of physical properties, classification skills, and inability to think abstractly.

4. The answer is B.

Hierarchical classification refers to the ability to understand the relationship between subordinate and superordinate classes. Matrix classification skills are more complex. Children can categorize things along 2 dimensions simultaneously, for example, baseball team by position. A 2-by-2 matrix would consist of 2 rows of teams (Red Sox and Yankees) and 2 columns of positions (pitchers and catchers). The matrix can expand or be rearranged to include multiple teams, positions, years, and players.

5. The answer is A.

Sternberg recognized that intelligence reflects the context in which it is embedded. That is, different cultures value different skills and place a greater premium on them.

6. The answer is D.

Gardner believed that we can no longer view intelligence as a unitary concept. Rather, different tasks require different intelligences.

7. The answer is B.

The DUPE model offers people several clear guidelines for solving problems in a logical manner.

8. The answer is B.

No one should be forced to use a technique with which they are uncomfortable. Both children and adults, depending on their personality and experience, will determine what is best for them.

9. The answer is C.

Kohlberg relied on moral dilemmas to discover the level of a person's moral development. This method forced subjects to indicate why they thought as they did.

10. The answer is D.

Gilligan believed that Kohlberg's dependence on male subjects neglected women's viewpoints. She argued that women traveled a different path of moral development.

11. The answer is A.

LEP stands for limited English proficiency. With the great wave of immigration that has swept the country, many children have difficulty with English.

12. The answer is B.

Controversy rages concerning the most effective means of teaching LEP students. Bilingual education seems to be growing in favor.

13. The answer is C.

By age 10, the development of a 2nd-person perspective allows children to put themselves in the other person's shoes and experience things from their point of view. They expect that friends will do the same for them. Children realize that if they can hide feelings and thoughts, so can others; social appearances can be deceiving. Friendships expand beyond sharing activities to include sharing subjective experiences. Trust means child does not hurt his or her friend's feelings, that the child understands the desire to be liked and accepted. Consequently, hurting people's feelings is understood to be intentional. Being excluded is painful.

14. The answer is D.

The school-age years are the period of "playground politics" because children learn to negotiate the complex social structure of the peer group. There are different kinds of friends for different occasions, alliances shift, and secrets are kept. The rough and tumble play and physical aggression of early childhood give way to competitive games of mental and physical skill. School-age children are inflexible about the rules of competition because they are a civilized way of resolving conflict and keeping aggressive tendencies in check. Competition can foster the development of social, mental, and physical skills through friendly rivalry, but when the only goal is to win, competition fosters dominance behavior.

15. The answer is D.

A school's emphasis on academic success sets it apart from other similar schools that lack this emphasis. Other qualities are secondary to academic success.

16. The answer is A.

Michael Rutter's work is a widely quoted study of school success with far-reaching implications. Its major conclusion stressed the significance of instructional excellence and emphasis on academic success.

17. The answer is C.

Creative or divergent thinking is marked by a search for novel ideas and products. Creative individuals are not afraid to diverge from customary paths.

18. The answer is A.

Unless a person has knowledge of a subject, it is difficult, if not impossible, for him or her to engage in divergent thinking.

19. The answer is C.

Case histories of children who were subject to early deprivation tell us the sensitive period for language development can be extended to age 6 if followed by high-quality nurturing.

20. The answer is B.

Children who are resilient have good cognitive and social skills, and easy-going personalities. Families are cohesive, with a multigenerational network of family members and friends that provides structure, rules, and expectations. Resilient children come from communities in which there are adult-run church and school programs, and health clinics.

21. The answer is C.

Developmental disabilities represent alterations in the typical developmental sequence in 1 or more of 3 areas: motor, cognitive, and neurobehavior. Motor includes gross-motor, fine-motor, and visuomotor coordination. Cognitive includes central processing, problem solving, and language. Neurobehavior refers to self-help, self-regulatory, and social skills. This triangle of developmental disabilities is characterized by delay, and/or dissociation, and/or deviation from the norm.

22. The answer is D.

The definition of gifted has 3 intersecting parts: above-average IQ, high levels of creativity, and high levels of commitment to a task. Giftedness is manifested in academics, creative thinking, leadership, visual/performing arts, and psychomotor abilities. About 5% of children can be considered gifted, which should not be confused with precociousness.

PART VI
Adolescence

57 Puberty

Composite of the sexual maturity rating scale

Stage	Characteristic		
	Genital Development in Males	**Pubic-Hair Development in Males and Females**	**Breast Development in Females**
1	Testes, scrotum, and penis are about the same size and shape as in early childhood.	The vellus over the pubes is not further developed than over the abdominal wall; in other words, there is no pubic hair.	There is elevation of the papilla only.
2	Scrotum and testes are slightly enlarged. The skin of the scrotum is reddened and changed in texture. There is little or no enlargement of the penis at this stage.	There is sparse growth of long, slightly pigmented, tawny hair, straight or slightly curled, chiefly at the base of the penis or along the labia.	Breast bud stage. There is elevation of the breast and the papilla as a small mound. Areolar diameter is enlarged over that of stage 1.
3	Penis is slightly enlarged, at first mainly in length. Testes and scrotum are further enlarged than in stage 2.	The hair is considerably darker, coarser, and more curled. It spreads sparsely over the function of the pubes.	Breast and areola are both enlarged and elevated more than in stage 2 but with no separation of their contours.
4	Penis is further enlarged, with growth in breadth and development of glans. Testes and scrotum are further enlarged than in stage 3; scrotum skin is darker than in earlier stages.	Hair is now adult in type, but the area covered is still considerably smaller than in the adult. There is no spread to the medial surface of the thighs.	The areola and papilla form a secondary mound projecting above the contour of the breast.
5	Genitalia are adult in size and shape.	The hair is adult in quantity and type with distribution of the horizontal (or classically "feminine") pattern. Spread is to the medial surface of the thighs but not up the linea alba or elsewhere above the base of the inverse triangle.	Mature stage. The papilla projects but the areola is recessed to the general contour of the breast.

Adolescence is bounded by the beginning and end of puberty, the period of physical maturation of the reproductive organs. These borders are imprecise, because puberty occurs in stages over time, beginning at ages 10–12 (in girls) and ending at 18–20 (in boys). The physical changes of puberty underlie the cognitive, social, and emotional changes that have earned adolescence the reputation for being a tumultuous and bittersweet time of life.

The term *puberty* refers to sexual maturity, which in girls means the onset of menstruation and in boys is harder to define. Prepubescence is the 2-year period of preliminary changes that occur prior to the onset of puberty. Postpubescence extends another 2 years or so beyond puberty, during which time bone growth is completed and the reproductive organs become fully mature. The sequence of sexual maturation has been described by Tanner (1990), whose Sexual Maturity Rating Scale is used by health care providers to track the development of breasts in girls and of the penis and scrotum in boys (**Table**).

Sex Characteristics and Hormones

Puberty begins when the hypothalamus starts to produce gonadotropin-releasing hormone (GnRH), which is transported via the bloodstream to the pituitary gland. The pituitary gland releases luteinizing hormone (LH), which stimulates the production of sex hormones by the gonads (ovaries and testes) and other endocrine glands in both males and females. Primary sexual characteristics (i.e., maturation of the ovaries, breasts, uterus, penis, and testes) develop in the reproductive organs as a result of sex hormone production. Secondary sexual characteristics, such as development of facial, body, and pubic hair, deepening voice, and distribution of fat and muscle, accompany hormonal changes but are not directly involved in reproduction.

Male sex hormones, called *androgens*, are produced by the cells of Leydig in the testes. The principal androgen is testosterone. In the male fetus, testosterone is responsible for development of the male reproductive organs. At puberty, testosterone stimulates overall growth, including muscles, vocal cords, and body hair, in addition to maturation of the reproductive system. Semen production begins and the male is able to experience erection and ejaculation. Boys experience "wet dreams" when they ejaculate semen during sleep.

In females, GnRH also stimulates the release of follicle-stimulating hormone (FSH) from the pituitary. Together, FSH and LH are responsible for the production of female sex hormones, estrogen and progesterone, from the ovaries. Recall that a girl's ovaries attain their full complement of egg cells—about 2 million—during prenatal development. Puberty marks the beginning of the menstrual cycle, during which an egg cell matures and is released into the uterus, making it available for fertilization from male sperm.

The menstrual cycle, which averages about 28 days, is complex and highly regulated by hormones. The cycle begins on day 1 with the onset of the menstrual flow. The first 13 days are called the *follicular phase*, during which FSH stimulates the follicles in the ovary to develop. As 1 follicle becomes more dominant and begins to secrete estrogen, the egg cell it contains matures. The increase in estrogen causes the lining of the uterus to thicken, and triggers a surge of LH at about day 14. The follicle ruptures and the egg cell, called the *oocyte*, is released into the fallopian tubes. This event is *ovulation*.

The second half of the menstrual cycle, about days 14–28, is the *luteal phase*. The ruptured follicle collapses, forming the corpus luteum, which secretes progesterone and small amounts of estrogen. Progesterone causes the uterine lining to mature in preparation for implantation of a fertilized embryo, and it inhibits the production of FSH, which would trigger the beginning of a new cycle. If fertilization does not occur, the increase in progesterone from the corpus luteum also shuts down LH, which sustains the corpus luteum itself. As the corpus luteum begins to disintegrate and progesterone levels fall, FSH production is no longer inhibited, and begins anew. Without progesterone, the lining of the uterus cannot be sustained, and it is shed in the form of the menstrual flow. The cycle begins again.

Causes and Effects of the Timing of Puberty

The production of sex hormones and of GnRH in the hypothalamus is subject to influence by genetics, nutritional and health status, chronic stress, and environmental factors. Today, the average age at the onset of menstruation among North American girls is 12.5 years, compared to age 17 about 100 years ago. For boys, the average age of puberty is 14, down from almost age 16 of a century ago.

Earlier onset of puberty has been attributed to better nutrition, especially fat intake, and to increased exposure to natural and artificial light. The brain may interpret the increase in light as evidence of environmental changes that support the growth of the food supply. The female body responds to a drastic drop in body weight and fat by shutting down menstruation, regardless of whether the cause is famine, illness, excessive exercise, or anorexia nervosa. Males may also experience a drop in sperm production in response to undue stress or illness.

The timing of puberty has important social implications. Early-maturing girls and late-maturing boys have the most difficulty adjusting. Girls who begin puberty at age 10 or 11 are a year or more ahead of their female peers, and 3–4 years ahead of their average male peers. The difference in physical maturity highlights the greater discrepancy in social, emotional, and cognitive maturity.

The late-maturing male still looks like a boy at age 15 or 16. Late-maturing males have difficulty competing with their physically mature male peers both in sports and in the social arena, undermining their self-confidence. Ironically, the late-maturing male may eventually grow to be larger than his early-maturing male peers.

58 Health

Tobacco

Objective: Increase by 1 year the average age of first cigarette use from 11.6 years to 12.6 years.

Objective: Establish tobacco-free environments and include tobacco use prevention in the curricula of all schools, preferably as part of quality school health education. (Baseline 17% in 1989).

Objective: Reduce the initiation of cigarette smoking among children and youth so that no more than 15% are regular smokers by age 20, compared to 30% in 1989.

Alcohol and Drugs

Objective: *Reduce* the proportion of young people ages 12–17 *who have used* alcohol, marijuana, or cocaine in the past month, as follows:

Substance	Baseline 1989	Target 2000
Alcohol	25.2%	12.6%
Marijuana	6.4%	3.2%
Cocaine	1.1%	0.6%

Objective: *Increase* the proportion of high school seniors who *associate risk* of physical or psychological harm with the heavy use of alcohol (5+ drinks on 1 occasion), regular use of marijuana, and experimentation with cocaine.

Behavior	Baseline 1989	Target 2000
Heavy use of alcohol	44%	70%
Regular use of marijuana	77.5%	90%
Trying cocaine once/twice	54.9%	80%

Physical Fitness and Nutrition

Objective: *Increase* to 75% the proportion of children and adolescents who exercise for at least 20 minutes or more 3 days a week.

Objective: *Increase* to 90% the proportion of school lunches that are consistent with dietary principles.

The U.S. Department of Health and Human Services (1990) initiated a national health promotion and disease prevention campaign called *Healthy People 2000*. (*Healthy People 2010* is being developed.) Some of the objectives relevant to school-age children and adolescents are in the **Table**. *Healthy Students 2000* (Allensworth et al., 1996) outlines how these objectives can be realized through school health education programs. In 1995, the Centers for Disease Control and Prevention (1996) conducted a national Youth Risk Behavior Survey among over 10,000 students in grades 9–12.

Nutrition and Exercise

Boys have higher caloric needs than girls because boys have a greater proportion of lean body mass to adipose tissue. A rapidly growing athletic 15-year-old boy may need as many as 4,000 calories a day just to maintain his weight. An inactive 15-year-old girl, whose growth is almost completed, may need fewer than 2,000 calories a day in order to avoid gaining weight. Half of adult bone structure is deposited during adolescence, requiring 1,200 mg of calcium a day.

Only 27% of adolescents eat the 5 or more recommended servings of fresh fruits and vegetables in a 24-hour period, foods rich in calcium, iron, and vitamins. About 65% eat more than 2 servings of high-fat food each day. Boys (32%) eat more fruits and vegetables than girls (22.7%), but boys (50%) also eat more fat compared to girls (29%). Boys simply eat more food, although boys are less likely to consider themselves overweight (22%) than girls (33.6%).

About 63% of teens exercise vigorously at least 3 times a week, boys (74%) doing so more than girls (52%), and whites (67%) more than blacks (53%). Participation in exercise of any kind, and in team sports in particular, declines from 9th to 12th grade, as work and other activities begin to take precedence.

Overweight and sedentary teens are at greater risk for dying before the age of 70 from heart disease, stroke, and colon cancer than their leaner and more active peers. Efforts to reduce the risk for disease range from healthier school lunches and nutrition education to early screening for high blood pressure and cholesterol.

Smoking

Both incidence and frequency of smoking cigarettes increase as students get older. While 63.4% of 9th graders have tried cigarettes, 75.8% of 12th graders have done so; similarly, 9.6% of 9th graders smoke frequently, rising to 20.9% by 12th grade. While smoking has declined among boys, it has not among girls, who believe it helps them to control their weight. Girls who smoke are perceived as "fun-loving" while nonsmoking girls are "sensible."

The best predictors of smoking behavior are having parents and friends who smoke, with the influence of friends being greater earlier in adolescence than later. Advertisements, especially those that implicate smoking with thinness in women, also play a role. Education programs that warn students about the long-term risks of smoking have not been successful. Adolescents not inclined to change their current behavior based on information alone. Successful smoking prevention programs have combined information about the dangers of tobacco with efforts to improve social skills and change attitudes about the social merits of smoking.

Alcohol and Drugs

By 12th grade, 83% of students have had at least 1 alcoholic drink, and over half of high school seniors (56%) report using alcohol within the past month. Half (51%) of all students in grades 9–12 report having used alcohol at some time during the previous 30 days, with 32% indulging in binge drinking. Boys (36%) are more likely to engage in binge drinking than girls (28%).

Use of marijuana and other drugs is more prevalent among boys and Hispanic students than among girls, and white and black students. While 42% of students in grades 9–12 have tried marijuana, 28% of males have used it within the past month, compared to 22% of girls. Sixteen percent of Hispanic students have tried cocaine, compared to 6.5% of white students and 2% of black students.

Alcohol use is strongly associated with other unhealthy behaviors, such as use of drugs and tobacco. About 40% of 10th graders report riding in a car driven by a peer under the influence of drugs or alcohol. Teens who use alcohol and drugs become sexually active at an earlier age and have more partners than teens who don't use these substances regularly. Sex while under the influence of drugs and alcohol is usually unprotected, placing adolescents at risk for sexually transmitted diseases (STDs) and unwanted pregnancy.

Adolescent drug and alcohol problems are associated with erosions in social values, economic viability, and family structure. Risk factors include family history of alcoholism, low academic aspirations, and antisocial behavior or social isolation during childhood. Successful prevention programs target family, community, and peers.

59 Sexuality

A Contraceptive use

Method	Who	Use
Abstinence	Grade 9 (age 14)	36%
	Grade 12 (age 18)	25%
Condoms	All adolescent couples	54%
	Grade 9 (age 14)	63%
	Grade 12 (age 18)	50%
	Black students	66%
	White students	52.5%
	Hispanic students	44%
Birth control pills	All adolescent couples	17%
	Grade 9 (age 14)	11%
	Grade 12 (age 18)	25%
	White students	21%
	Black students	10%
	Hispanic students	11%

B Sexually transmitted diseases

Disease	Cause/symptoms/risks	Incidence
Chlamydia infection	Caused by microorganisms May be no symptoms Causes 20%–40% of female infertility	5–7 million new cases per year Black and Latino teens at higher risk
Gonorrhea	Caused by bacteria, skin-to-skin contact Painful urination Discharge from penis or vagina	1–2 million new cases per year 25% are teens
Genital herpes	Caused by virus, skin-to-skin contact No cure Open sores on the genitals	500,000 new cases per year 30 million people affected
HIV/AIDS	Caused by virus, primarily blood borne May be no symptoms No cure	Teens are new highest risk group

During adolescence, physical and social factors influence the development of a sexual identity that incorporates body image, feelings of sexual arousal, and choices regarding sexual behavior. Religion, marriage customs, and attitudes about the sexual roles of men and women set the cultural context in which adolescents come to terms with their sexual identities.

Developmental Challenges of Adolescent Sexuality

While it is normal to forge a sexual identity during the teen years, adolescent sexuality has often been viewed as a problem waiting to happen. Parents, health care providers, and educators warn teens about pregnancy, date rape, and sexually transmitted diseases (STDs). Less attention has been paid to how a healthy sexual identity develops. Brooks-Gunn and Paikoff (1993) proposed that adolescent sexual well-being is an integration of physical, social, cognitive, and emotional factors. They identify 4 developmental challenges.

Puberty and Body Image

The first challenge occurs with the onset of puberty. Girls who develop early and boys who develop late are most unhappy with their bodies, and feel less attractive to the opposite sex. Satisfaction with body image is also influenced by cultural norms. American girls are particularly self-conscious about their weight. Boys want to be athletic and muscular.

Managing Sexual Arousal

The second challenge is the management of sexual arousal. It is normal to be flooded with desire, and yet teens receive mixed messages about how to deal with their feelings. Boys are most readily aroused by visual stimuli, hence their interest in sexually explicit magazines. Sexual arousal in girls, however, is not as openly acknowledged. It may also be more complex. While girls are attracted to handsome boys, being the object of male desire also makes girls feel sexy. Overt displays of sexuality in girls, and discussion of their desires, remain taboo.

Sexual Behavior

The third developmental challenge involves sexual behavior. Studies of college freshmen indicate that while about 45% of males masturbate once or twice a week, 47% of females report they never masturbate (Jones and Barlow, 1990). Heterosexual behavior refers to sexual interactions with the opposite sex, from hand holding to intercourse. Homosexuality refers to a sexual preference for members of one's own sex. Adolescents need to learn how to negotiate sexual situations so that they do not engage in risky sexual behaviors.

Safe Sex

The fourth challenge is to avoid the unnecessary risks of pregnancy and STDs by practicing safe sex or by abstaining from intercourse (see **Parts A** and **B**) (Centers for Disease Control and Prevention, 1996).

Sexual Behavior

Dating is a new phenomenon. In many cultures, the onset of puberty was accompanied by mating rituals. Today, especially in industrialized countries, a decade or more separates the onset of puberty and marriage. Teenagers must wrestle with critical questions: How much petting is okay? Do I have intercourse before marriage or not? Should a girl carry condoms? American culture has not helped them. Teenagers are bombarded by messages that promote sexuality without restraint or responsibility.

In 1971, only 14% of 15-year-old girls and 26% of 17-year-old girls had experienced sexual intercourse. By 1990, those numbers were 43% and 66%, respectively. By age 18, 73% of males are no longer virgins. Girls are more likely to approve of intercourse when it is part of an exclusive love relationship, but 24% admit they gave in to pressure from boyfriends the first time. Only 20% of girls found their first experience to be pleasurable, with 34% reporting it was "a disaster" or "a disappointment" (Dacey and Kenny, 1997).

Boys not only expect physical intimacy earlier in a dating relationship, but also overestimate the sexual activity of their male peers. Boys engage in first coitus because they perceived the girl wanted to (19%), because they were curious (18.6%) or aroused (18%), or because they cared for the girl (18%). About 52% found the first experience to be "terrific" or "pleasurable."

Teens who come from stable families in which parents demonstrate responsible behavior and are open to discussing sex with their children are less likely to engage in premarital sex. Those who do are older at first coitus. Teens whose families are poor, disorganized, and endorse the view that women are subservient to male dominance become sexually active at an earlier age (Forste and Heaton, 1988). Similar factors influence the use of contraceptives (see **Part A**) and incidence of teen pregnancy.

Teenage Pregnancy

About 1 million teenage girls become pregnant each year; more than half (530,000) give birth. Nearly 13% of all babies born in the United States in 1991 were born to teens (National Center for Health Statistics, 1993), 62 per 1,000 (U.S. Bureau of the Census, 1994). Sadly, 1 in 3 teenage mothers drops out of school.

60 Cognitive Development

A   Cognitive Development in Adolescence

- Thinking applies to possibilities as well as the realistic.
- Thinking relates to the future as well as the present.
- Thinking is evident in hypothetical-deductive statements.
- Thinking demonstrates logical reasoning.
- Thinking illustrates the use of abstract concepts.

B

- Ability to consider possibilities.
- Ability to consider alternatives.
- Ability to engage in propositional thinking.
- Ability to combine pertinent facts.
- Ability to apply concrete data.
- Ability to acquire needed data.
- Ability to improve existing competencies.

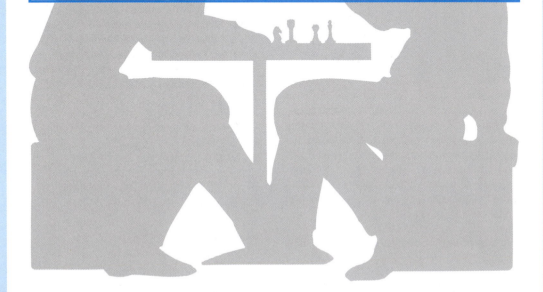

150

Piaget's stage of formal operations is a fruitful beginning for any analysis of adolescent thought. According to Piaget, the *formal operational* period, during which the beginnings of logical, abstract thinking appear, commences at about the age of 11 or 12 years.

Piaget's Stage of Formal Operations

During adolescence and the appearance of formal operations, youngsters demonstrate an ability to reason realistically about the future and to consider possibilities that they actually doubt. Teenagers look for relations, they separate the real from the possible, they test their mental solutions to problems, and they feel comfortable with verbal statements. In short, the period's great achievement is a release from the restrictions of the tangible and the concrete (Elkind, 1994) (see **Table**).

Some adolescents, however, may still be in the concrete operational stage, or only into the initial stages of formal operations. They have just consolidated their concrete operational thinking and continue to use it consistently. Unless they find themselves in situations that demand formal operational thinking (such as science and math classes), they continue to be concrete operational thinkers. As Elkind (1994, p. 221) noted, learning how to use formal operations takes time and practice with a blend of concrete and abstract materials.

Features of the Formal Operational Period

There are several essential features of formal operational thinking:

1. *The ability to separate the real from the possible*, which distinguishes the formal operational thinker from the concrete operational thinker. Adolescents try to discern all possible relations in any situation or problem and then, by mental experimentation and logical analysis, attempt to discover which are true.
2. *Adolescent thinking is propositional*, which means that adolescents use not only concrete data, but also statements or propositions that contain the concrete data. Dealing with abstract concepts no longer frustrates them. Also, their increasing ability to deal with "If this . . . then that" statements may cause them to argue more vigorously about any controversial matter such as drug use, school programs on sexual conduct, or political issues.
3. *Adolescents attack a problem by gathering as much information as possible and then making all the possible combinations of the variables that they can.* They proceed as follows: *First*, they organize data by concrete operational techniques (classification, seriation). *Second*, they use the results of concrete

operational techniques to form statements or propositions. *Third*, they combine as many of these propositions as possible. *Fourth*, they then test to determine which combinations are true.

Other Characteristics of Adolescent Thought

Flavell, Miller, and Miller (1993) identified several other features of adolescent thought:

- **An increase in domain-specific knowledge.** Adolescents simply have accumulated more knowledge in many subjects than have younger children.
- **Greater information-processing capacity.** Development seems to be the key explanation here. The speed of information processing increases and leads to an expansion of functional capacity.
- **Advances in metacognition.** "Thinking about thinking" becomes an important part of adolescent thought. Children gradually acquire knowledge about cognitive functioning, that is, how people process information.
- **Improvement of existing competencies.** Adolescent thought is distinguished not only by the acquisition of new abilities (e.g., propositional thinking), but also by an improvement in the competencies already possessed (see **Tables**).

Implications for Health Care Providers

The adolescent years are a time of rapid change. If you find yourself dealing with teenagers, learn as much as possible about all aspects of adolescent development. In most cases, adolescents retain the fears of a child when faced with the consequences of an accident or disease. Yet, simultaneously, they try to muster the bravado that these years demand. Be honest, and answer questions as fully as possible. Don't hesitate to ask direct questions: Are you using birth control pills? Listen carefully to their answers and don't dismiss any warning signs as "typical teenage talk." Too often throwaway statements such as "I'd like to kill myself" have turned out to be tragically prophetic.

When working with adolescents, be careful not to exaggerate their abilities. Observe their reactions as they answer your questions or describe symptoms. Keep in mind the features of formal operational thought:

- Can they separate the real from the possible? Some adolescents will still have a difficult time.
- Are they comfortable with propositional thinking?
- Can they help you gather as much data as needed and combine clues, thus helping you to make vital decisions?

Adolescent Thought

Characteristics of adolescent thought

Characteristic	Explanation and Implication
Egocentric thinking	Thinking more about one's self than about others. Adolescents become self-absorbed.
Imaginary audience	Thinking everyone is looking at one's self. Adolescents are painfully self-conscious.
Personal fable	Seeing one's self as unique and powerful. Adolescents' belief in their abilities is inflated.
Social cognition	The ability to think about interpersonal relationships, to make sense of other people's behavior. Adolescents learn to manipulate the rules of social engagement.
Second-person perspective	The ability to see an event from someone else's point of view. Adolescents understand exclusion from the group is deliberate and intended to be hurtful.
Third-person perspective	The ability to observe one's self playing out a role in a social situation in relationship to others. Adolescents scrutinize themselves.
Betrayal	When an understanding between 2 parties is violated. Adolescents feel betrayed when they act in accordance with what they think are the rules of a relationship, and find that the other party did not.
Disillusionment	When an established social schema is proved false. Adolescents learn their idols have flaws.

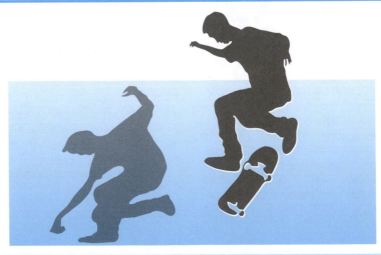

Adolescents can think abstractly. Younger adolescents appreciate that symbols can represent reality, such as the use of metaphor in poetry. Older adolescents manipulate systems of symbols. They appreciate themes in literature and discuss complex ideas, such as justice. Adolescents' ability to reason becomes more systematic. They use hypothetical reasoning to ask, "What if?" This approach to problem solving is akin to the scientific method.

The emergence of abstract thinking has several important implications for social and psychological development (see **Table**). Elkind (1984) referred to the increased complexity of cognitive processing during adolescence as "thinking in a new key."

Egocentric Thinking: Imaginary Audience and Personal Fable

Adolescents spend a lot of time thinking, and thinking about their thinking. They tend to see themselves not as others see them but as they think others must see them. Being absorbed in their own experience, adolescents think that others think they are unique and fascinating, or awful and stupid.

Egocentric thinking results in what Elkind called the "imaginary audience" and the "personal fable." Younger adolescents in particular are extremely self-conscious (Selman and Schultz, 1991), sure that everybody is looking at them. They perform for an audience that exists in their imaginations, and use it to anticipate the reactions of other people to their behavior.

Adolescents also feel different from everyone else. Believing that they are unique means that others—especially those older than them—cannot understand their thoughts and feelings. If adolescents are alone in their experience, they also need to perceive themselves as all powerful and indestructible. The personal fable enables adolescents to create stories in which they are capable of great and important things. Adolescents also appreciate and deny their own mortality. Personal fables afford adolescents the opportunity to play with alternate social scenarios mentally, and can sharpen social cognitive abilities.

Social Cognition and Perspective Taking

There are 2 aspects of social cognition (Fiske and Taylor, 1984): social schemas and how they change. *Social schemas* are mental representations of the role that people play in different situations and relationships. Schemas are based on personal experiences and how people organize them. They change with experience and maturity.

Perspective taking influences social cognition and the development of schemas (Selman and Schultz, 1991). When older children and young adolescents take a second-person perspective, they see an event from someone else's point of view. This gives them some insight into others' intentions and feelings. The third-person perspective refers to the ability of older adolescents to step outside of themselves, and watch how they play out their role in different situations. It is related to later abstract thinking, when adolescents can think in terms of interactions within and between systems.

Both types of perspective taking challenge existing social schemas. Adolescents understand that exclusion from the group is intended to be deliberate and hurtful. They see that some groups are more open to new membership than others. Members of a group learn to jockey for position. Adolescents also discover that girls and boys approach relationships with different expectations. Teens learn the strategic manipulations of social survival. Those who misunderstand the rules, and those who follow the rules when others do not, feel betrayed and disillusioned.

Adolescents become disillusioned when they realize their idols have flaws. The "Big Man on Campus" is shallow; the admired teacher has a drinking problem. In time and with maturity, adolescents use the third-person perspective to scrutinize themselves. They relinquish the personal fable and replace it with more realistic, yet still idealized, expectations. The importance of the imaginary audience fades, and adolescents begin to develop their own set of standards to guide their behavior. Changing social schemas can lead to greater self-understanding in the adolescents who can negotiate the emotional discomfort that such psychological and social adjustments entail.

Argument and Debate

Adolescents appreciate the art and science of debate. They approach problems systematically, collect the relevant facts, find the logic in them, and make their case with passion, and an unshakable belief they are right. They love to exercise their new cognitive abilities, and to outmaneuver opponents with carefully crafted strategies. That is, adolescents argue for the sake of arguing.

As painful as adolescent argumentativeness is for adults, it can help teenagers sharpen their cognitive and social skills. Once adults recognize argument as a form of mental exercise, they can help adolescents to argue constructively, to focus on the principles under discussion and to defuse the emotion.

Implications for Health Care Providers

Adolescence is probably the most difficult time to have serious health problems. The excessive attention to one's physical health feeds into their self-centeredness and self-consciousness. Adolescents may correctly perceive themselves as different from peers. The very real threat to mortality challenges personal fables about invulnerability. The ability to live in one's mind means that "just thinking" about illness is stressful. The frustration and anger associated with the illness experience, added to their natural tendency to argue, can make life difficult for them and the people who care for them (Thies and Walsh, 1999).

Peer Relationships

A Do parents know what their teens are doing?

Do you think that your child...	Parental myth	Teen reality
Has contemplated suicide?	9%	26%
Has cheated on a test?	37%	76%
Has had sex?	9%	19%
Has friends with drug problems?	12%	36%
Has driven a car while drunk?	22%	46%

B Interpersonal understanding and peers

Level	Friends	Peers	Adults
Level 0 (3–6 yr) Undifferentiated and egocentric	Friendship depends on physical closeness.	A physical activity holds group together (playing with toys).	Authority figures.
Level 1 (5–9 yr) Differentiated and subjective	Someone who does what child wants.	Unilateral relations; little perspective of others.	Caretakers and helpers.
Level 2 (7–12 yr) Looks at self objectively; realizes others can do what they want	Interactions become desirable in themselves.	Values relationships.	Counselors
Level 3 (10–15 yr) Complex concept of people; may have mixed feelings about same person	Mutual interests and sharing.	Sees group as social whole.	Tolerated; mutual satisfaction begins to develop.
Level 4 (12+ yr) Understands complexity of individuals and relationships	Different relationships satisfy different needs.	Begins to understand group dynamics.	Interactions begin to change.

The importance and the influence of peers in development cannot be exaggerated. In the 1940s, Anna Freud (Sigmund Freud's daughter) and Sophie Dann worked with 6 German-Jewish orphans whose parents had died in the Nazi gas chambers. The 6 children spent several years together in a concentration camp, enduring horrible conditions, with few adult contacts. When the war ended, the children were taken to England to recover. Although they showed some effects of their ordeal—thumb sucking, fearfulness, restlessness—they were strongly attached to each other, to the point where they comforted each other when disturbed and became upset when separated. With the loving care that the children received over the subsequent years, coupled with their continued relationships with their peers, they gradually showed normal patterns of development (Freud and Dann, 1951).

The Meaning of *Peer*

We typically use the word *peer* to refer to those who are similar in age, usually within 12 months of each other. But equal in age does not mean equal in everything, for example, intelligence, physical ability, or social skills. Also, research shows that many interactions are with those who are more than 12 months older.

Most adolescents still want to remain close to parents, but the tugs of separation and independence are powerful, leading to strains in the home. The attraction of peer relationships grows intense and assumes a sensitivity and sense of belongingness that challenges adults to remain "sensitively responsive."

Adolescents whose parents were warm, responsive, and consistent disciplinarians are more competent with peers than those whose parents are harsh and rejecting or overly permissive (**Part A**).

Teenagers are acutely aware they must get along with peers, which forces them to think about their relationships, a major step in social development. For example, they begin to make definite judgments about the behavior of their peers and become more astute at detecting meaning in facial expressions and in the way something is said. Their increasing social skills and cognitive maturity enable them to recognize that other points of view exist.

Social Perspective Taking

Selman (1980) believed that people's views on relationships cannot be separated from their personal theories about the psychological characteristics of others. Selman identified several levels of social perspective taking and noted that youngsters gradually comprehend that other people are different and have ideas of their own. As they move into adolescence, their views of a relationship include self, someone else, and the kind of relationship between them. The desire to conform now becomes achingly important. Selman's 5-level analysis of interpersonal understanding is illustrated in **Part B**.

The Formation of Peer Groups

The view of adolescence has changed in recent years. Although the adolescent period brings challenges, anxiety, excitement, and even upsets, for most adolescents it is not a time of great stress, turmoil, and trouble (Lerner and Galambos, 1998). More frequently than not, the peer group becomes a positive force during these years and exercises many positive functions.

Tracing the changes in the nature of peer groups from childhood to adolescence, Brown (1990) noted the following:

- Adolescents spend much more time with their peers than do children, and during high school spend twice as much time with peers as with parents and adults.
- Adolescent peer groups receive much less adult supervision than do groups of children.
- More frequent interactions with peers of the opposite sex occur as time with parents decreases.
- Adolescents typically tend to identify with a particular group (sports, drama, music, adventure seekers).

Biological, psychological, and social changes in adolescence occur simultaneously and can cause considerable anxiety and insecurity (Lerner and Galambos, 1998). Thus turning to others who share the same experiences is a natural inclination for most teenagers. Their dependence on parents lessens, and their dependence on their peers increases.

Implications for Health Care Providers

Working with teenagers can be both frustrating and fulfilling, frustrating in that they feel they must maintain the appearance of independence and fulfilling because if you gain their confidence, you can accomplish so much. Remembering the adolescent characteristics discussed in this chapter will help you to develop and maintain good relationships with them.

Keep in mind that adolescents are capable of abstract thought, so explain the current situation clearly and also the consequences of the condition that brought the adolescent to you. Try to capitalize on adolescents' relationships with their peers by urging them to discuss their condition with their friends, who may have experienced a similar problem.

63 The Search for Identity

A Erikson and the search for identity

Age: 12–18 years

Stage: Adolescence

Psychosocial crisis: Identity versus identity confusion

Psychosocial strength: Fidelity

Environmental influence: Peers

B Identity status

	Diffusion	Foreclosure	Moratorium	Achievement
Crisis	absent	absent	present	present
Commitment	absent	present	absent	present
Period of adolescence	early	middle	middle	late

For many years adolescence had been thought of as a time of tremendous turmoil. Recently, however, theorists and researchers have concluded that upset and turmoil are not the defining characteristics of adolescence. Rather, most adolescents adjust to the socialization demands of family, school, and society. They have also acquired friends who, for the most part, share these values. But the process of passing through these years introduces a certain tension for all adolescents, particularly with regard to their identity.

Identity or Doubt

The adolescent years, from about ages 12–18, have come to be identified with Erikson's colorful description of them as the time of "identity versus identity confusion." Recall (see Chapter 2) that Erikson believed personality development occurred through a series of conflicts, both inner and outer, and that individuals emerge from each crisis with a greater sense of inner unity, an increase in good judgment, and a growing tendency to live by personally significant standards.

Erikson viewed the adolescent years as the end of childhood and the beginning of adulthood. Teenagers display an acute sensitivity about what others think of them, and peer opinion now plays a large part in how they think of themselves. If uncertainty at this time results in *identity confusion*, a bewildered youth may withdraw, run away, or turn to drugs. Youngsters faced with the question "Who am I?" may be unable to answer. The challenges are new; the tasks are difficult; the alternatives are bewildering. Needless to say, adults must have patience and understanding.

Identity versus Identity Confusion

Faced with a combination of physical, sexual, and cognitive changes, joined with heightened adult expectations and peer pressure, adolescents understandably feel insecure about themselves—who they are and where they are going. By the end of adolescence, those who have resolved their personal crises have achieved a sense of identity. They know who they are. Those who remain locked in doubt and insecurity experience what Erikson calls *identity confusion*. Erikson's views on identity have generated considerable speculation, theorizing, and research (**Part A**).

For example, Marcia (1966, 1980) concluded from a series of studies that adolescents seem to respond to the need to make choices about their identity (particularly regarding career, religion, or politics) in one of 4 ways:

1. **Identity diffusion,** or the inability to commit one's self; the lack of a sense of direction. Adolescents experiencing identity diffusion lack a cohesive, consistent whole; they simply lack a genuine identity of their own.

2. **Identity foreclosure,** or making a commitment only because someone else has prescribed a particular choice; being "outer-directed." That is, they have not identified and resolved a crisis, but have accepted the dictates, usually of parents, about the direction of their lives.

3. **Identity moratorium,** or the desire to make a choice at some time in the future but being unable to do so. These adolescents are actively grappling with an identity crisis, but as yet have not resolved it.

4. **Identity achievement,** or the ability to commit one's self to choices about identity and maintaining that commitment under all conditions.

Part B summarizes Marcia's views on identity status.

Helping Adolescents Find Their Identity

Adults can help adolescents acquire psychosocial maturity by adopting the following suggestions:

- **Treat them as almost adult;** that is, provide them with independence, freedom, and respect.
- **Challenge them with realistic goals** that coordinate their activities with college and career choices.
- **Use ideas that challenge, not defeat,** and that are both biologically and psychologically appropriate.
- **Constantly address the issue of identity versus identity diffusion.** For example, parents and teachers can help adolescents discover their strengths and weaknesses through their classroom work.
- **Parents and teachers should work together,** and teachers should be encouraged to have their students write a journal entry about anything they wish. Many will write about personal problems. After all the entries are submitted, teachers can write answers to their questions and comments on the information in the entries.
- **Stress the skill of communication both at home and at school.** By being able to express how they feel in groups and with individuals and by learning how to listen, teenagers will realize that they are not the only ones who are confused.

Implications for Health Care Providers

Today's adolescents are maturing in a time of social turbulence in their life spans. Sex, drugs, alcohol, personal relationships, career choices, and interactions with parents pose daily challenges to adolescents.

Probably the most important strategy to remember in working with teenagers is to treat them as "almost adults." Listen—really listen—to them. Don't talk down to them. Rather explain in clear, nonemotional terms the nature and dimensions of the problem they brought to you. This may be the crisis that crystalizes the adolescent's sense of identity.

64 Motivating Adolescents

A Motivation — theories and themes

Theorist	Theory	Theme	Key Idea
Maslow	Humanistic	Needs hierarchy	Need satisfaction
Bruner	Cognitive	Intrinsic processes	Mixed motives
Weiner	Attribution	Causes of behavior	Perceived causes of behavior
Skinner	Behaviorism	Reinforcement	Schedules of reinforcement
Bandura	Social cognitive	Observation	Modeling

B

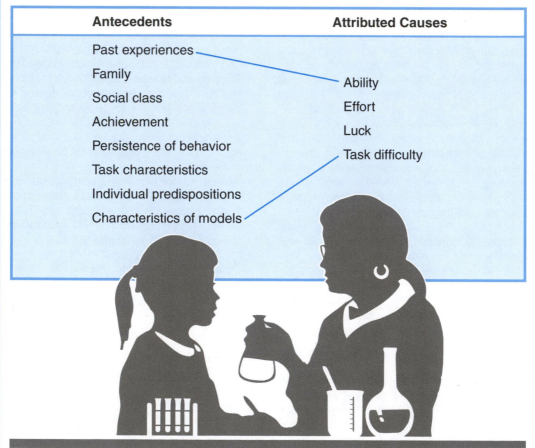

Antecedents	Attributed Causes
Past experiences	Ability
Family	Effort
Social class	Luck
Achievement	Task difficulty
Persistence of behavior	
Task characteristics	
Individual predispositions	
Characteristics of models	

People who set their sights on realistic goals and believe they have the ability to reach them have taken a major step on the roadway to success. This is as true for adolescents as any other age group. Determination, positive attitude, and feelings of competence contribute powerfully to academic achievement, good relations with others, and positive interactions with parents, teachers, and other adults. One of the most significant psychological contributors to successful passage through adolescence is motivation.

The Meaning of *Motivation*

When people ask about motivation, their intent is usually to discover what causes people to act in a particular way, what their inner feelings about their situation are, and what they want—what their goal is. It is difficult to specify just what motivation is, but a good, working definition is as follows: *Motivation arouses, sustains, directs, and integrates behavior.*

Another way of coming to grips with the meaning of motivation is to examine several motivational theories (**Part A**). (Here we recommend that you review Chapter 6.)

Cognitive Psychology and Motivation

Cognitive theorists believe that internal processes, such as thinking, control human behavior. Jerome Bruner (1966), one of the leading cognitive theorists of this century, believed that there is an ideal level of arousal between apathy and wild excitement.

Bruner turned to the notion of *discovery* as a means of furthering intrinsic motivation. Arguing that discovery leads to new insights, Bruner believed that people learn to manipulate their environment more actively and achieve considerable gratification from personally coping with problems.

Attribution Theory and Motivation

All people attribute their behavior to a specific cause, and these attributions then serve as a guide to their expectations for future success or failure. *Attribution theory* rests on 3 basic assumptions (Weiner, 1980): *First*, people want to know the causes of their own behavior and that of others. *Second*, people do not randomly assign causes to their behavior. They assume there is a logical explanation for the causes to which they attribute their behavior. *Third*, the causes that people assign to their behavior influence subsequent behavior.

Individuals tend to attribute their performance to 1 of 4 elements:

1. **Ability.** Adolescents' assumptions about their abilities are usually based on past experience, and when they have a history of failure, they often make the devastating assumption that they lack ability.
2. **Effort.** Adolescents (like all humans) judge their efforts by how well they did on a particular task.

3. **Task difficulty.** Task difficulty usually is judged by the performance of others on the task. If many succeed, the task is perceived as easy, and vice versa. If individuals consistently succeed on a task at which others fail, they will attribute success to ability. But if their success is matched by the success of others, then the source of the success is seen in the task (it was easy).
4. **Luck.** Finally, if there is no tangible link between behavior and goal attainment, the tendency is to attribute success to luck.

Behavioral Psychology and Motivation

One of the great behaviorists of our time, B. F. Skinner (1971) stated that if you ask people why they go to the theater and they reply that they feel like going, you are usually satisfied. It would be more revealing, however, if you knew what happened when they previously attended the theater, what they had read about the play, and what else induced them to go.

According to Skinner, if adolescents obtain reinforcement for certain behavior, they tend to repeat it with vigor. If they do not obtain reinforcement, they tend to lose interest and their performance suffers.

Bandura and Social Cognitive Learning

Albert Bandura's social learning theory has particular relevance for motivation, since he believed that an important impression is made on adolescents not by telling them what to do, but by setting an example for them. When this happens, they also begin to develop a sense of self-efficacy, which Bandura (1997, p. 3) defined as belief in one's capabilities to organize and execute the courses of action required to produce given attainments.

Implications for Health Care Providers

One of your major concerns in working with adolescents should be their psychological reaction to their condition. For example, adolescents are highly sensitive about their self-image. Anything threatening their view of themselves will affect their willingness to cooperate with you, and may even affect the rate and extent of their recovery.

An eclectic approach to teenagers would seem to be the best solution. For example, whenever possible, reinforce any positive efforts they make, such as faithfully doing prescribed exercises, or taking medication as scheduled. Encourage them to think about the reasons why they came to see you so that they see themselves as personally involved in planning what is needed to correct the condition. Perhaps, most importantly, help them to develop a sense of personal efficacy in their efforts to recover. Once they feel confident in their ability to succeed in whatever program you design for them, they will have a much greater chance of regaining their health.

65 Delinquency

Delinquency

Home	**School**	**Personal**
Poor Parenting Behavior	Disruptive	Low IQ
Emotional Instability	Conduct Disorder	Self-assertive
Criminality	Fighting	Defiant
Family Discord	Hostility	Aggressive
Broken Home	Poor Achievement	Impulsive

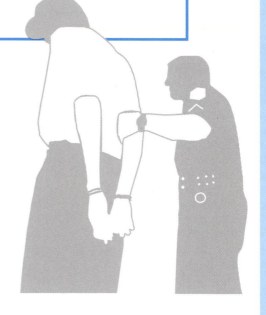

Increasing violence in our society has focused attention on juvenile delinquency, youth gangs, random aggression, and drug use. Although most youths never become involved with law enforcement agencies, the extent of youth crime and violence cannot be ignored (see **Table**).

Think of *delinquency* as behavior that the public at any specific time thinks is in conflict with its best interests. (This definition thus includes behavior that is personally nonadaptive and legally sanctioned.) The causes of delinquency defy easy categorization. Usually it is difficult to identify just what propelled a boy or girl along the troubled path to delinquency. One of the most disturbing characteristics of juvenile crime is its increasing tendency toward violence.

The Roots of Delinquency

In their massive study of crime and human nature, Wilson and Herrnstein (1985) found clear evidence of a positive association between past and future antisocial behavior; that is, the best predictor of violence is past antisocial behavior. Although the causes of violent and criminal behavior are multiple and complex, most modern scientists believe that a tendency to commit crime is established early in life, *perhaps as soon as the preschool years*, and that the behaviors of these children provide ample clues to their possible future antisocial behavior.

A critical age for early signs of emerging delinquency is 7–12 years when children search for friends and want to become accepted members of a group, some of which encourage antisocial acts. They may be drawn to a particular group because a friend is a member; it may be a sign of rebellion (my mother doesn't like those kids, but I think they're neat); or it may just seem a daring thing to do.

The Characteristics of Delinquents

In their lifelong studies, the Gluecks (1950) found that delinquents were distinguishable from nondelinquents in several ways:

- **Physically.** They were more muscular and vigorous.
- **Temperamentally.** They were restless, energetic, impulsive, extroverted, aggressive, and destructive.
- **Attitudinally.** They were hostile, defiant, resentful, and stubborn, and resented authority.
- **Psychologically.** They were more interested in the concrete than the abstract and had no strategies for solving problems.
- **Socioculturally.** They were more often reared in homes that offered little understanding, affection, stability, or moral standards.

More recent studies reached similar conclusions:

- There may be something *genetic* at work; for example, both members of identical twin pairs are more likely to be involved in delinquency than are nonidentical twins.
- *Males* are more prone to criminal behavior than females, and younger males are more likely to commit crimes at a higher rate than older males.
- *Attitudinally*, most children prone to behavior problems are hostile, defiant, resentful, and suspicious, and resistant to authority (Regoli and Hewitt, 1991).
- *Psychologically*, delinquents are more interested in the concrete than the abstract and are generally poor problem solvers (Travers et al., 1993).
- *Socioculturally*, delinquents are frequently reared in homes that offer little understanding, affection, stability, or moral clarity.

Controlling Impulsive Behavior

Impulsivity seems to be a continuous thread running through delinquent behavior. Studying impulsivity, researchers placed children in a position in which they were presented with something they enjoy—candies, toys—and were told if they do not eat the candy or play with the toy until the researcher returns, they can have 2 pieces of candy or an even bigger toy. The researcher then left the room and observers watched the children through 1-way mirrors. The results were as one would expect: Some children ate the candy immediately or played with the toy; others resisted by trying to distract themselves.

The amazing part of this work, however, was the follow-up research. The same children who displayed impulsivity at age 4 years were the more troubled adolescents: They had fewer friends; they experienced more psychological difficulties such as lower self-esteem; and they were more irritable and aggressive, more prone to delinquent behavior, and less able to cope with frustration. The 4-year-olds who delayed their gratification could better handle frustration, were more focused and calm when challenged by any obstacle, and were more self-reliant and popular as adolescents.

Implications for Health Care Providers

Be alert to the signs of the major risk behaviors: drug and alcohol abuse, unsafe sex and teenage pregnancy, school underachievement, and delinquency, crime, and violence (Lerner and Galambos, 1998). Remember also that many adolescents are desperate for recognition and acceptance. Finally, become familiar with community programs that are designed to help troubled adolescents and recognize the diverse development of children and adolescents.

66 Mental Health Problems

A   Criteria for major depressive disorder, single episode

A. Five or more of the following symptoms have been present during the same 2-week period and represent a change from previous functioning. At least 1 symptom is either (1) depressed mood or (2) loss of interest or pleasure.

    (1) Depressed mood; in adolescents can be irritable mood

    (2) Diminished interest or pleasure in all or almost all activities

    (3) Significant weight loss without dieting or weight gain (e.g., 5% in a month)

    (4) Insomnia or hypersomnia every day

    (5) Psychomotor agitation or retardation nearly every day

    (6) Fatigue or loss of energy nearly every day

    (7) Feelings of worthlessness or excessive or inappropriate guilt nearly every day

    (8) Diminished ability to think or concentrate, or indecisiveness, nearly every day

    (9) Recurrent thoughts of death, recurrent suicidal ideation without specific plan, or a suicide attempt or specific plan for committing suicide

B. Symptoms do not meet criteria for Mixed Episode (i.e., depressive and manic symptoms)

C. Symptoms cause significant distress or impairment in social, occupational, or other areas of functioning.

D. Symptoms are not due to the physiological effects of a substance or medical condition.

E. Symptoms are not accounted for by Bereavement.

B   Warning signs for possible suicide in adolescents

1. Talking about killing oneself "I wish I were dead." "My family would be better off without me."

2. Preoccupation with death, in music, art, poetry, personal writings; talking about "not being" or not having a future: "I have nothing to live for." "It won't get any better so what's the use."

3. Disturbances in eating or sleeping habits.

4. Declining grades in school, lack of interest in school or hobbies.

5. Giving away prized possessions.

6. Withdrawal from family and friends, feeling alienated from others.

7. Significant changes in usual behavior or demeanor, e.g., the shy person becomes an extravert.

8. Series of "accidents" or impulsive risk-taking activities.

9. Pervasive sense of gloom, hoplessness, helplessness.

Teens comprise an age group that many consider at risk for depression simply by virtue of their developmental period. Normative changes may be accompanied by dissatisfaction with body type, disappointment in love, uncertainty about the future, anxiety about sexuality, and conflict with family. For some, however, feelings of despair and hopelessness are out of proportion to developmental events. When that happens, the risk for suicide increases.

Characteristics and Incidence of Depression in Adolescence

The **Table** lists the criteria for a diagnosis of major depression according to the *Diagnostic and Statistical Manual of Mental Disorders*, 4th edition (1994). *Social/emotional symptoms* include dejected mood, loss of pleasure, social withdrawal, and crying spells. *Physical symptoms* include fatigue, sleep disturbance, and loss of appetite. *Cognitive symptoms* include difficulty concentrating, indecisiveness, and distorted perceptions about events and relationships. Cognitive difficulties may result in poor academic performance. Teens may withdraw into sleep, television, or video games.

The incidence of depression increases steadily through the teen years. About 20%–35% of teens experience mild depression at some point. Another 10%–15% experience moderate depression, while 5% are severely depressed (Brooks-Gunn and Petersen, 1991). Moderate and severe depression are not simply "more depression" than mild symptoms. Major depression represents a significant and negative alteration in how individuals think about themselves, their future, and life experiences. That is, major depression can become self-sustaining, shaping future experiences.

Risk Factors for Depression

Risk factors for depression in adolescence include significant loss, health problems, family history, abuse, and alcohol use. Loss can be the death of a loved one, rejection in love, or dashed hopes and dream. Teens with serious health problems are 2.5 times more likely than healthy peers to experience significant depression and anxiety (Wallander and Varni, 1992). A history of abuse, especially sexual abuse, and a family history of depression, especially in a parent, increase risk. Adolescents who use drugs or alcohol are also more likely to suffer from depression. The lack of perceived emotional and social support magnifies risk factors.

Girls are at greater risk for depression than boys, although the suicide rate among boys is higher. Girls are more likely to be dissatisfied with their body type and to blame themselves for their failures. They feel responsible for maintaining relationships, and may experience a greater sense of loss and failure when things do not work out as expected. Girls internalize their feelings and ruminate over negative experiences and feelings. Boys blame others or bad luck for their failures. They externalize their feelings, expressing them with action and often with aggression.

Suicide and Adolescents

Depending on the source, either suicide or homicide is the second leading cause of death between ages 15 and 24, with accidents ranked number 1.

The suicide rate for white males aged 15–19 increased between 1970 and 1990 from about 8 to 20 per 100,000. For nonwhite males, the rate increased from about 6 to 13 per 100,000 in the same time period. Suicide rates among adolescent females, by contrast, have been more steady. Among nonwhite females, the rate dropped between 1970 and 1990, from about 3 to 2.5 per 100,000, whereas it rose from 3 to 4 per 100,000 among white adolescent girls aged 15–19.

According to a 1995 survey by the Centers for Disease Control and Prevention, about 30% of female high school students have thought seriously about attempting suicide, compared to 18% of male students. Girls were also twice as likely as boys to make an attempt (12% vs 5.6%). However, boys are 5 times more likely to die by suicide than are girls. Girls are more likely to use an overdose of pills or alcohol, or both, whereas boys resort to more violent and lethal methods, such as firearms and hanging. Boys who commit suicide may be more emotionally disturbed than girls, and more determined to die. However, use of firearms among girls is increasing. While 6% of teens report they have attempted suicide, 15% report having considered it seriously. About 60% of American teenagers know someone who has attempted suicide.

Risk Factors for Suicide

Risk factors for suicide include a history of emotional or psychiatric disturbance, especially affective disorders, such as depression and bipolar disorder. Adolescent girls who commit suicide are also more likely to suffer from borderline personality disorder, whereas boys manifest antisocial and conduct disorders. Adolescents who die from suicide have histories that include early and frequent use of alcohol and other substances, especially cocaine, and early and frequent sexual activity. Among males in particular, concerns about homosexuality is a risk factor for suicide.

The comorbidity of alcohol use and emotional disorder, especially coupled with sexual acting out, are powerful predictors of suicidal behavior. However, the best predictor is a previous attempt. Almost 50% of adolescents who die by suicide made a previous attempt. **Part B** lists the warning signs for possible suicide in adolescents.

PART VI: QUESTIONS

Directions: For each of the following questions, choose the **one best** answer.

1. Which of the following is an example of secondary sexual characteristics?

(A) Onset of menstruation in girls

(B) Growth of breasts in girls

(C) "Wet dreams" in boys

(D) Growth of facial hair in boys

2. Which hormone is responsible for the onset of menstrual flow?

(A) Estrogen

(B) Progesterone

(C) Follicle-stimulating hormone (FSH)

(D) Luteinizing hormone (LH)

3. What are the caloric needs of a rapidly growing adolescent boy?

(A) 1,500 calories per day

(B) 2,000 calories per day

(C) 3,000 calories per day

(D) 4,000 calories per day

4. Which of the following has the greatest influence on adolescents' decision to smoke cigarettes?

(A) Advertisements showing celebrities smoking

(B) Having parents who smoke

(C) Having friends who smoke

(D) Having good social skills

5. Who among the following is apt to be least happy with their bodies?

(A) Early-maturing boys and early-maturing girls

(B) Early-maturing girls and late-maturing boys

(C) Late-maturing boys and late-maturing girls

(D) Late-maturing girls and early-maturing boys

6. Which of the following factors is most influential in adolescents' decision to become sexually active?

(A) Their family environment

(B) Difficulty managing sexual arousal

(C) The values depicted in the media

(D) Peer pressure

7. An ability to think about the future and consider negative possibilities is a feature of Piaget's

(A) sensorimotor period.

(B) preoperational period.

(C) concrete operational period.

(D) formal operational period.

8. Adolescents demonstrate an increase in

(A) searching ability.

(B) information-processing capacity.

(C) classroom sophistication.

(D) unilateral methodology.

9. A young adolescent refuses to walk through the mall with his mother, saying he's old enough to take care of himself in a public place. According to Elkind, this is an example of

(A) the imaginary audience.

(B) the personal fable.

(C) the second-person perspective.

(D) social cognition.

10. Why do adolescents argue so much?

(A) They like to argue.

(B) They are capable of propositional reasoning.

(C) They enjoy outmaneuvering their opponents.

(D) All of the above are correct.

11. When adolescents want to do something themselves, this is an example of

(A) persistence.

(B) logical processing.

(C) internal motivation.

(D) search and discovery.

12. People tend to attribute their performance to ability, effort, task difficulty, or

(A) luck.

(B) influence.

(C) diligence.

(D) peers.

13. *Peer* usually refers to those who are within _____ months of each other.

(A) 10

(B) 12

(C) 18

(D) 24

14. The work of _____ is associated with social perspective taking.

(A) Selman

(B) Skinner

(C) Vygotsky

(D) Freud

15. Erikson's famous term for what adolescents may experience is

(A) discovery crisis.

(B) assimilated identity.

(C) structured ego.

(D) identity crisis.

16. The expression "adolescent egocentric thinking" is associated with

(A) Piaget.

(B) Marcia.

(C) Bruner.

(D) Elkind.

17. One of the most disturbing features of today's delinquency is its increasing

(A) spread.

(B) violence.

(C) hidden nature.

(D) family directedness.

18. Delay of gratification studies attempt to identify _____ children.

(A) impulsive

(B) delayed

(C) emotionally disturbed

(D) aggressive

19. Depression affects 3 major areas of functioning in adolescents. Which of the following are examples of symptoms in those areas?

(A) Crying, loss of pleasure, social withdrawal

(B) Fatigue, weight loss, trouble sleeping

(C) Drop in grades, cannot think straight, cannot make decisions

(D) Loss of pleasure, sleep disturbance, difficulty concentrating

20. What is the best predictor of suicide among adolescents?

(A) Psychiatric disorder

(B) Abuse of alcohol and drugs

(C) Early sexual activity

(D) A previous attempt

PART VI: ANSWERS AND EXPLANATIONS

1. The answer is D.

Primary sexual characteristics involve the reproductive organs as a result of sex hormone production, i.e., maturation of the ovaries, breasts, uterus, penis, and testes. Secondary sexual characteristics accompany hormonal changes but are not directly involved in reproduction; these include development of facial, body, and pubic hair; deepening voice; and distribution of fat and muscle.

2. The answer is B.

Progesterone causes the uterine lining to mature in preparation for implantation of a fertilized embryo, and it inhibits the production of FSH, which would trigger the beginning of a new cycle. If fertilization does not occur, the increase in progesterone from the corpus luteum also shuts down LH, which sustains the corpus luteum itself. As the corpus luteum begins to disintegrate and progesterone levels fall, FSH production is no longer inhibited, and begins anew. Without progesterone, the lining of the uterus cannot be sustained, and it is shed in the form of the menstrual flow. The cycle begins again.

3. The answer is D.

Boys have higher caloric needs than girls because boys have a greater proportion of lean body mass to adipose tissue. A rapidly growing, athletic, 15-year-old boy may need as many as 4,000 calories a day just to maintain his weight. An inactive 15-year-old girl whose growth is almost completed may need fewer than 2,000 calories a day to avoid gaining weight.

4. The answer is B.

The best predictor of smoking behavior is having parents who smoke. The influence of friends is greater earlier in adolescence than later. Advertisements, especially those that implicate smoking with thinness in women, also play a role. Adolescents who are socially skilled are more self-confident, and less likely to succumb to the influence of peers to engage in risky behaviors.

5. The answer is B.

The timing of puberty can have a significant impact on how adolescents feel about their new bodies. Girls who develop early and boys who develop late are most unhappy with their bodies, and feel less attractive to the opposite sex. Early-maturing girls are self-conscious about their bodies, and subject to teasing from boys who typically develop later than the average girl. Late-maturing boys appear to be boys among the women and young men in their class, and have more difficulty competing in athletics and socially.

6. The answer is A.

Of the many factors that influence adolescents' choice to become sexually active, the family environment is the most significant. Teens who come from stable families in which parents demonstrate responsible behavior and are open to discussing sex with their children are less likely to engage in premarital sex. Those who do are older at first coitus. Teens whose families are poor, disorganized, and endorse the view that women are subservient to male dominance become sexually active at an earlier age. Adolescent girls who have goals for their future involving education and career also delay first coitus.

7. The answer is D.

Reversibility and ability to speculate about things that seem impossible help to identify formal operational thinking.

8. The answer is B.

Most adolescents acquire a greater ability to process data than they had as children. For example, they usually can store greater amounts of information in memory.

9. The answer is A.

Egocentric thinking results in what Elkind calls the "imaginary audience." Younger adolescents in particular are extremely self-conscious, sure that everybody is looking at them. Hence, they may act as if on stage, performing for an audience that exists in their imaginations. They may use the audience to anticipate the reactions of other people to their own behavior.

10. The answer is D.

Adolescents argue for the sake of arguing. Propositional reasoning, that is, analyzing the logic of propositions, means adolescents appreciate the art and science of debate. They approach problems systematically, collect the relevant facts, find the logic in them, and make their case. They invest the presentation of their case with passion, and an unshakable belief they are in the right. They love to exercise their new cognitive abilities, to see different perspectives, to discuss abstract principles, to analyze the intentions that underlie behavior, and to outmaneuver opponents with carefully crafted strategies.

11. The answer is C.

Individuals who want to do something themselves do not need external rewards such as praise, recognition, or anything tangible. They are driven by a desire to accomplish a particular task, to excel, to discover.

12. The answer is A.

Individuals who believe luck is the basis of any success they achieve typically lack self-esteem. They believe that control is out of their hands.

13. The answer is B.

Interestingly, although 12 months is thought of as the age criterion for a peer, many relationships are formed on the basis of mutual interests and likes or dislikes.

14. The answer is A.

The significance of Selman's work lies in its insights into psychosocial development. When children and adolescents begin to realize that others have their own opinions and ideas, it affects how they relate to those around them.

15. The answer is D.

Teenagers who are uncertain as to their own self (i.e., identity crisis) have difficulty in resolving the personal crises that accompany these years.

16. The answer is D.

Elkind's expression aptly captures the egocentrism of adolescence. Besieged by physical and emotional changes, adolescents tend to think that everything revolves around them.

17. The answer is B.

Those concerned with the delinquency problem are alarmed at the growing violence. Whether due to changed societal conditions, a breakdown in authority, or televised aggression, new kinds of intervention are needed.

18. The answer is A.

Research showing how impulsivity is linked to achievement demonstrates its importance in all phases of development.

19. The answer is D.

The criteria for depression address 3 major areas of functioning. *Social/emotional symptoms* include dejected mood, loss of pleasure, social withdrawal, and crying spells. Depressed individuals lose interest in the routines of daily living. *Physical symptoms* include fatigue, sleep disturbance, and loss of appetite. *Cognitive symptoms* include difficulty concentrating, indecisiveness, and distorted perceptions about events and relationships.

20. The answer is A.

The comorbidity of alcohol use and emotional disorder, especially coupled with sexual acting out, are powerful predictors of suicidal behavior. However, the best predictor is a previous attempt. Almost 50% of adolescents who die by suicide made a previous attempt.

PART VII
Adulthood

67 Early Adulthood: Physical Health

A Rate of decline in organ reserve

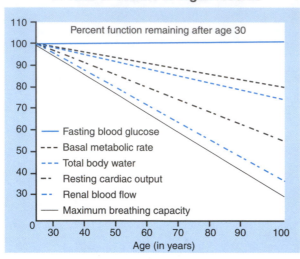

Percent function remaining after age 30

- —— Fasting blood glucose
- ---- Basal metabolic rate
- ---- Total body water
- -·-· Resting cardiac output
- -·-· Renal blood flow
- —— Maximum breathing capacity

Age (in years)

B The health practices associated with good health

Eat breakfast almost every day

Rarely or never eat between meals

Sleep 7–8 hours daily

Maintain normal weight adjusted for height, age, and sex

Never smoke cigarettes

Avoid alcohol or use it moderately

Engage in regular physical activity

C Health promotion model

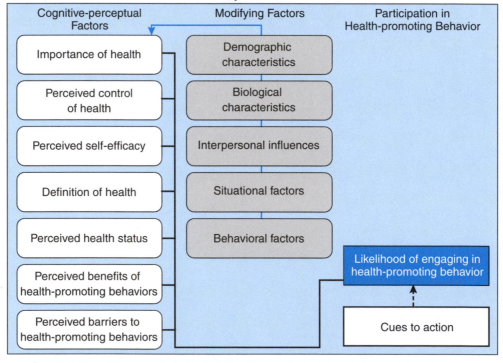

Cognitive-perceptual Factors	Modifying Factors	Participation in Health-promoting Behavior
Importance of health	Demographic characteristics	
Perceived control of health	Biological characteristics	
Perceived self-efficacy	Interpersonal influences	
Definition of health	Situational factors	
Perceived health status	Behavioral factors	
Perceived benefits of health-promoting behaviors		Likelihood of engaging in health-promoting behavior
Perceived barriers to health-promoting behaviors		Cues to action

Source: Pender, N. (1996). Health promotion in nursing practice. Norwalk, CT: Appleton & Lange.

Humans are at the peak of physical development and performance between ages 20 and 30. The built-in reserve of vital capacity in major organs and biological systems remains robust until about age 30, after which there are varying rates of decline (see **Part A**). The health habits that develop during this period are excellent predictors of how humans will weather the physical changes and diseases that typically emerge in the middle and later years. **Part B** lists the 7 health habits most closely associated with good health.

Characteristics of Biological Systems

Body Mass, Height, and Weight
The average American woman is 5 feet 4 inches tall, and reaches that height by about age 18. Men reach the average height of 5 feet 9 inches at about age 20. A weight gain of 10–15 lb between ages 18 and 30 is largely due to the maturing of muscles, bones, and internal organs and an increase in fatty tissue. Overindulgence in food and alcohol, is the major reason for obesity during this period.

Skin, Hair, and Teeth
As total body water begins to decrease, and time spent in the sun accumulates, skin becomes drier. Male pattern balding, which begins with hair loss at the crown and is genetically determined, begins in the 20s and 30s. Wisdom teeth often causes problems that lead to their removal.

Musculoskeletal System
Fusion of the epiphyses of the long bones occurs between ages 18 and 25, which is also the peak of muscle performance. After age 26, muscle strength begins to decline and reaction time levels off. Declines in muscle mass and body water content may be masked by increase in fatty tissue, giving a false impression of vigor. Decline in water content in the joints results in small skeletal changes after age 30, increasing vulnerability to knee, ankle, and shoulder injuries.

Cardiovascular and Pulmonary Systems
The heart and lungs can achieve 100% capacity when required to do so during the 20s. Following age 30, the rate of decline depends on activity level and smoking status. The risk for heart and lung diseases in middle age depends largely on the choices made in youth. The long-term effects of smoking, lack of exercise, a diet high in fat, and overuse of alcohol are the major contributors to heart disease and stroke (see Chapter 66).

Reproduction
Pregnancy and childbirth are major physical events for women in their 20s and 30s. Fertility rates decline and the incidence of birth defects and complications during labor rise after age 30. Pregnancy results in multiple changes in all body systems. Blood volume and cardiac output increase 25%–50% and oxygen consumption increases 20%. The residual volume of the lungs decreases by 20%. Fatigue and shortness of breath are not uncommon. As the uterus increases in size, it displaces the stomach and intestines, leading to heartburn and constipation. Toward the end of pregnancy, the pelvic ligaments and joints soften to facilitate birth, but cause difficulty walking. Most women benefit from moderate exercise throughout pregnancy.

Health Promotion
Primary prevention refers to efforts to prevent disease and injury in healthy people. Examples include immunizations, use of seat belts, and self-breast examinations. Health promotion is directed at increasing one's well-being, in part through healthy lifestyle choices. The U.S. Department of Health and Human Services in its *Healthy People 2000* initiative has identified its top 4 priority areas for health promotion and disease prevention as physical activity and fitness, nutrition, tobacco use, and alcohol use. Other areas include mental health, family planning, and violence.

Young adulthood is prime time for establishing good health habits. The Health Belief Model addresses the relationship between health and behavior (Rosenstoch, 1974). The first and second components of the model are perception of susceptibility to a particular illness and perception of the seriousness of the illness. The third component is weighing the costs and benefits of taking preventive action.

For example, if your father died of heart disease at age 55 and you are 45 years old, a smoker, and overweight, you perceive yourself to be susceptible to a serious disease in the near future. The perceived benefits of losing weight and quitting smoking outweigh your costs in time, money, and aggravation. If you have no personal experience with heart disease and are under age 30, you do not perceive yourself as being susceptible. The hassle of watching your diet and giving up cigarettes outweigh the perceived benefits.

The Health Promotion Model (Pender, 1996) (see **Part C**) addresses the likelihood of choosing to adopt health-enhancing behaviors. Cognitive perceptual factors include perception of how healthy one is, how much control one has over health, whether one thinks one is capable of changing habits, and the benefits of healthy behaviors. These are modified by factors such as age, interpersonal influences, social group, and education. For example, if you want to lose weight, but believe you have inherited your weight problem, you do not perceive yourself to be in control of your health, and are less likely to change your eating habits.

68 Early Adulthood: Cognitive Development

A Traits characterizing intelligence at various ages

6-month-olds	Recognition of people and objects Motor coordination Alertness Awareness of environment Verbalization
2-year-olds	Verbal ability Learning ability Awareness of people and environment Motor coordination Curiosity
10-year-olds	Verbal ability Learning ability, problem solving, reasoning Problem solving Reasoning Creativity
Adults	Reasoning Verbal ability Problem solving Learning ability Creativity

B

Piaget	——	Formal Operational Thinking
Perry	——	Rigidity - Flexibility - Commitment
Schaie	——	Achieving stage (applying knowledge)

Three transformations occur in the shift from adolescence to early adulthood.

1. The structure of thought changes as young adults, using the foundation of earlier cognitive development, turn to distinct ways of thinking.
2. Young adults concentrate on acquiring advanced knowledge in a particular field as they begin their careers.
3. The path of intellectual development may remain relatively stable or decline sharply during the adult years.

The Transition to Adult Thinking

One of the major features of adult thinking, beginning in adolescence and becoming more firmly rooted in early adulthood, is the tendency to analyze verbal statements and to evaluate their validity as formal propositions (Flavell et al., 1993).

When faced with a problem, adults immediately search for possibilities. They examine the situation carefully, look for all possible solutions, and then analyze them to determine which is the best possible answer. They follow the steps of scientific reasoning. (See Chapter 45 for a discussion of problem solving.)

Another outstanding feature of adult thought is the acquisition of specific knowledge combined with a greater capacity for information processing. Both these features plus speed and accuracy contribute to the reasoning abilities needed in problem solving. With improvement in memory, for example, adults solve problems more readily by remembering similar problems and how they were solved.

Explanations of Adult Thought

Several theories have been proposed to explain changes in adult thinking. Piaget's final stage of formal operations represents his interpretation of adolescent and adult thought. Piaget believed that there are several essential features of formal operational thinking:

- **Individuals at this stage of cognitive development can separate the real from the possible.** They try to identify all possible relations in any problem and then, by mental experimentation and logical analysis, discover which are true.
- **Formal operational thinking is propositional,** which means that individuals can use statements and propositions to reach conclusions.
- **Formal operational thinkers attack a problem by gathering all available information and then combining as many variables as possible.**

Among the theorists who concentrated on adult cognitive development was William Perry (1970, 1981), who interviewed 67 Harvard and Radcliffe students at the end of each of their 4 years of college and discovered several important ways in which the thinking of young adults differs from that of adolescents. As younger students, they held rigid ideas about right and wrong, good and bad. This rigid, dualistic thinking gradually grew more flexible, however, when they began to realize that their opinions on many matters were as good as those of others. As they continued to accumulate knowledge and to better understand how their values affect their thinking, the young adults made their own commitments. That is, they reached their own decisions and committed to their own beliefs, while simultaneously accepting that other valid possibilities exist. As you evaluate Perry's ideas and assess their universality, remember that his subjects were taken from a small, highly select and educated group.

Another explanation of cognitive development in early adulthood was proposed by K. Warner Schaie (1977; Schaie and Willis, 1992). Schaie believed that young adults differ from adolescents in the way that they *use* their cognitive abilities. The problems they encounter become more complex; the situations they face become more diverse; the decisions they make become more critical. Although young adults continue to acquire knowledge in specific, more restricted fields, their cognitive focus shifts more to the application of knowledge.

Schaie formulated several stages to trace and explain adult cognition. He termed the early adult stage the *achieving* stage to indicate how young adults apply their cognitive abilities to those circumstances that have profound long-term consequences, such as career, marriage, and family (see **Part B**).

Implications for Health Care Providers

Young adults are relatively healthy, which means that you need to be insightful and creative in suggesting care for this age group. Because they possess the cognitive abilities described in this chapter, they are more likely to comprehend treatment procedures you recommend. You will contact many individuals in this age group on college and university campuses. Consequently, try to advocate programs stressing positive health behaviors, perhaps in courses with a health education component or in peer counseling groups. Identify as many opportunities as possible for health promotion and protection in places where young adults gather.

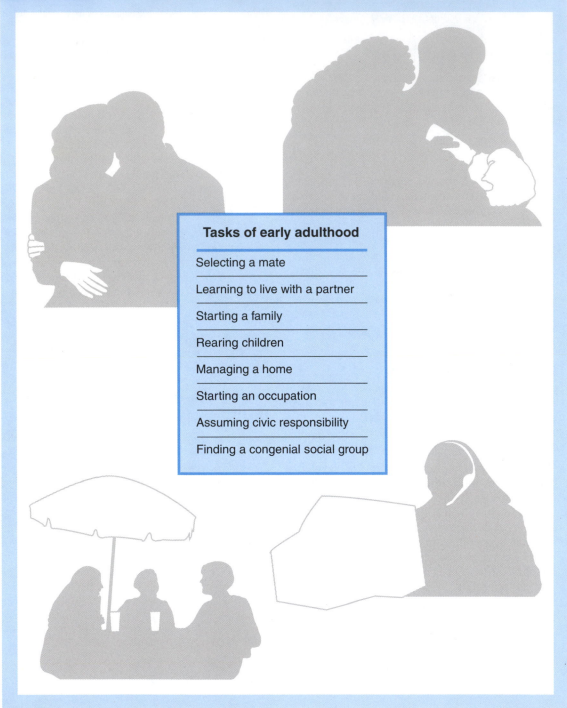

69 Early Adulthood: Psychosocial Development

Tasks of early adulthood

Selecting a mate

Learning to live with a partner

Starting a family

Rearing children

Managing a home

Starting an occupation

Assuming civic responsibility

Finding a congenial social group

The early adult years are often described as a "time of firsts": job, marriage, pregnancy, children, education of children, owning a home. It is a testing period for any 1 or 2 individuals; they are now relatively independent, free to make their own mistakes. Psychiatrist George Valliant (1993), well-known chronicler of the life span, referred to the "two anxieties" of the early adult years: commitment to another person, and success in a chosen career.

Intimacy and Isolation

Erik Erikson's interpretation of the early adult years is found in stage 6 of the life cycle, *intimacy versus isolation*, that is, a person's intimate commitment to another.

Positive intimacy implies being with another person in an interdependent, committed, and intimate manner while simultaneously retaining a needed core of independence. Reconciling these 2 opposites leads to the basic conflict of Erikson's stage 6. Resolving the crisis of this stage depends on both internal (a person's capacity for love) and external (one's partner) influences.

During these years, an identity crisis may reemerge as the struggle to resolve the independent-interdependent conflict. Without resolution, a person may define himself or herself through his or her partner, thus sacrificing self-esteem and initiative. A person who has achieved intimacy with another, however, transfers a sense of ease to other relationships, yet is perfectly fine when alone.

The Seasons of a Person's Life

Believing that there are 4 major seasons of life, Yale psychologist Daniel Levinson conducted 2 famous studies on life spans, one of men in 1978 and the other of women in 1996. A key concept in Levinson's work is the notion of life structure, that is, the basic pattern or design of a person's life at any given time. Life structure is whatever a person finds important—another person, an institution, an occupation—and for most people, life structure is built around family and work. Levinson believed that men in the early adulthood years face several major tasks:

- During these years, men develop a dream or vision that sparks vitality and provides motivation and energy for the tasks that lie ahead. For most men, the dream involves career choices and a blueprint detailing the road to success in their chosen occupations.
- Formulating a dream is tied tightly to a relationship with a mentor who is usually an older colleague, although occasionally a friend or relative may serve the role.
- During these years, men select a partner and determine the nature and quality of the relationship with that person.

At about age 30, men typically go through a transition period where they question the quality of their lives—their life structures—and speculate on ways to improve it. During the later years of the early adult period, men focus on consolidating their careers, establishing harmonious family relationships, and becoming more involved in community affairs.

Women's path through these years, while similar, nevertheless has a different timetable. *Gender splitting* (rigid divisions separating men and women) has declined due to changed thinking about women's role in a modern society. As a result of widely adopted birth control techniques and a high divorce rate, the idea of a female homemaker and a male provider is no longer the standard for family life.

Adapting to Life

In 1938, two physicians at Harvard University, Arlie Bock and Clark Heath, received a grant from philanthropist William T. Grant to study healthy human lives. Two hundred sixty-eight sophomores were selected for study and followed for 30 years. (Only 20 of the subjects dropped out over the course of the study.) Thirty years later, George Valliant interviewed the subjects when they were 47 years old, inquiring about their work, families, and physical and psychological health.

He described a typical developmental path for most of the men: During their 20s and 30s, they established their independence from their parents and began their own families. Sometime in their 30s and 40s, after achieving a desired intimacy with a partner, they entered a stage of career consolidation; that is, they clearly defined their career choices and goals characterized by commitment, compensation, contentment, and competence. As Valliant (1993) noted, these 4 words distinguish a career from a job.

Implications for Health Care Providers

The early adult years are typically a time of good health. However, more and more young adults are becoming increasingly aware of the preventive benefits of a good diet, exercise, and regular checkups. Consequently, positive health behaviors, safety practices, diet, exercise, sexuality, addiction, and stress are widely discussed topics among today's young adults.

You should be alert to opportunities to encourage practices designed to prolong these years of good health. Colleges and universities are natural settings for lectures, seminars, and health fairs that both encourage and inform. In business settings, topics such as nutrition, stress management, blood pressure monitoring, smoking reduction, and employee relationships are among subjects suited for workers.

70 Middle Adulthood: Physical Health

A Cardiovascular disease and stroke: risk factors

Risk Factor	Explanation of Risk
Smoking[a]	Damaged lungs ⟶ poor oxygen exchange ⟶ less oxygen to major systems ⟶ increased workload on heart + hypertension
Hypertension[a] > 160/90 mm Hg	Decreased elasticity of blood vessels ⟶ increased workload on Heart + impaired blood flow to brain (⟶ stroke) and impaired blood flow to heart muscle (⟶ myocardial infarction)
Diabetes (type I)[a]	High blood glucose ⟶ chronic damage to blood vessels ⟶ increased risk of peripheral vascular disease ⟶ impaired blood flow to and from extremities via the heart and lungs
High cholesterol Total > 200 mg/dL LDL > 180 mg/dL	Increased plaque ⟶ narrowed diameter of arteries + clots in arteries + damage to blood vessel interior wall ⟶ hypertension + increased workload on heart + impaired blood flow to heart muscle (⟶ myocardial infarction) and to brain (⟶ stroke)
Obesity	Diet high in fats + less physical activity ⟶ increased workload of heart + increased risk for diabetes and hypertension
Stress	Increases heart rate and blood pressure, liver releases cholesterol and fatty acids into bloodstream
Alcohol overuse	Empty calories + poor dietary habits + lack of exercise ⟶ elevates arterial blood pressure ⟶ overload on heart

Note: LDL = low-density lipoprotein.　　[a]Indicates major risk fact ors according to the Framingham Heart Study.

B Decision tree for the treatment and management of menopause

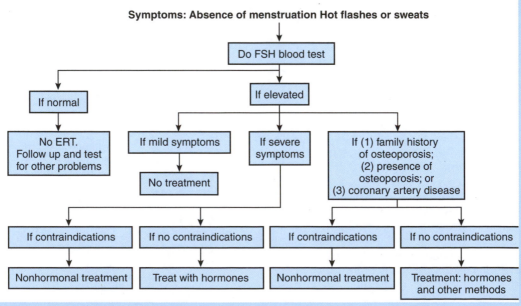

Symptoms: Absence of menstruation Hot flashes or sweats

The Aging Process

Nature brings life from conception to the peak of reproductive capacity. After that, there is no genetic plan for maintenance. Life runs on reserve power (see Chapter 63). Aging is not a disease, although the incidence of disease increases with age, and disease can make people age more quickly.

Stochastic theories propose that aging events are random, cumulative, and microscopic. For example, random exposure to radiation can cause mutations in DNA, causing cells to malfunction. The slow accumulation of damage to cell membranes by free radicals (the by-products of oxygen metabolism) is another stochastic theory. The free radical theory is related to the cross-link, or connective tissue, theory. It proposes that chemical reactions bind molecular structures that work best when separate, such as proteins, nucleic acid, and collagen. These structures change the composition of soft tissue, such as skin, muscles, and blood vessels, compromising their effectiveness. Nonstochastic theories propose that aging is genetically programmed into the lives of cells. For example, a genetic timetable shuts down the ovaries, causing menopause.

Age-Related Changes

Weight
The ratio of lean body mass to fat decreases with time. As the metabolic needs of lean tissue are greater than those of fat, metabolic needs decrease during midlife. Adults who do not compensate by eating fewer calories and less fat and by increasing exercise will gain weight.

Skin, Hair, and Teeth
Exposure to sunlight, specifically ultraviolet rays, may hasten the normative overgrowth of elastin and loss of collagen in the dermis, the layer of skin beneath the epidermis. Wrinkles and sagging occur when the subcutaneous layer of connective tissue and fat shifts.

Hair is given its color by melanin, which is produced by cells called melanocytes in hair follicles. When these cells wear out during midlife, they are not replaced. Hair loses its color and appears gray or white.

Periodontal disease first appears in midlife, first as gingivitis. Plaque irritates the gums, making them tender, inflamed, and more likely to bleed. As plaque builds up, gums begin to recede from the teeth and open spaces appear between the teeth (periodontitis). Eventually, teeth become loose and the gums infected. Good oral hygiene is the best preventive measure.

Vision and Hearing
The need for reading glasses is a definitive marker of middle age. The lens within the eye thickens and the eyeball elongates. Refracted images fall short of the retina, and objects within 18 inches or so of the eye are out of focus, a condition called *presbyopia*. *Presbycusis* refers to a decreased ability to hear the higher frequencies (3,000–4,000 hertz). Adults in midlife occasionally miss consonant sounds found in this higher range. "Bed," "bet," and "vet," sound alike, especially against background noise.

Musculoskeletal Changes
By midlife, there is some loss of bone mass and muscle fibers as cells wear out and are not replaced. The water content of cartilage decreases, as does the manufacture of synovial fluid in joints. With less lubrication, joints, especially the knees, stiffen. The rate of decline in strength and endurance varies greatly among individuals. Inactivity, nutrition, and disease rather than aging alone account for the rate of decline.

Cardiovascular Changes
Cells in the heart and diaphragm, 2 muscles in constant use, do not change much with age. However, elastic properties of the heart and blood vessels are altered by other factors, related largely to diet, smoking, and inactivity. Fat and connective tissue infiltrate muscle and nerve cells in the heart and narrow arteries. Poorly oxygenated blood further starves the heart muscle. The decrease in the flow of oxygenated blood to the heart muscle, alterations in electrical conduction within the heart muscle, and the inefficiency of infiltrated muscle cells in the heart valves all compromise the heart's functioning.

Cardiovascular disease (CVD) is the leading cause of death among adults in the United States. Since 1948, the Framingham Heart Study has monitored thousands of male and female volunteers leading to the identification of the major risks factors for CVD, and the role of diet, exercise, and stress in the development and prevention of heart disease and stroke (see **Part A**). In 1991, the National Institutes of Health began the Women's Health Initiative to study CVD in postmenopausal women.

The incidence of CVD is the same in women as in men, except that women develop the disease about 10 years later than men. Women seem to be protected against CVD by an "estrogen umbrella" prior to menopause. After menopause, their risk for CVD and osteoporosis increases, sparking the debate about the value of hormone replacement therapy for women in midlife.

Reproductive Changes
Menopause is the most significant physical change in women at midlife (review Chapter 53). The symptoms associated with menopause are related to the rate of decline in estrogen production. The faster the drop off, the more severe the symptoms, such as heavy bleeding, hot flashes, night sweats, insomnia, and irritability. Women who have been heavy smokers reach menopause earlier, and may have a sharper decline in estrogen than nonsmokers. **Part B** is a decision tree for the treatment and management of menopause with estrogen replacement therapy (ERT).

Middle Adulthood: Cognitive Development

Cognitive development in middle adulthood

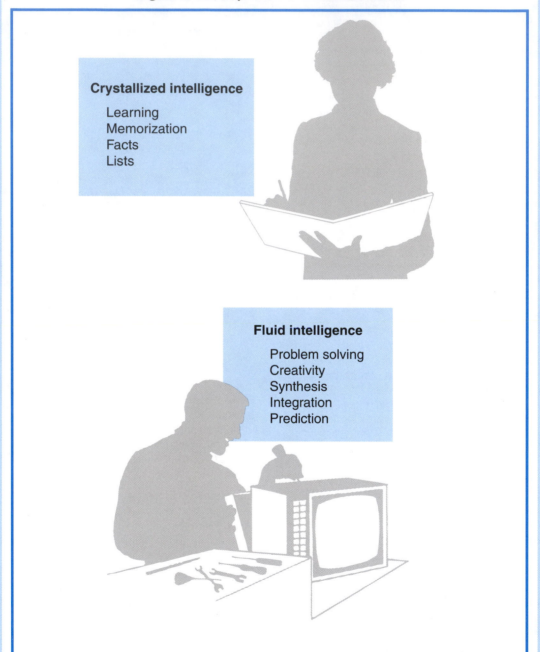

Crystallized intelligence

Learning
Memorization
Facts
Lists

Fluid intelligence

Problem solving
Creativity
Synthesis
Integration
Prediction

During these years, most men and women reach the peak of their influence in their careers, in their families, and in the community. At the same time they have established an intimate bond with a partner or have taken steps to repair or resolve a troubled relationship. Physical changes during these years (increased risks of cardiac problems for men, breast cancer for women) lead to periods of self-evaluation, even self-doubt. Simultaneously, external pressures—career demands, family obligations, care of aging parents—increase, causing many middle-aged adults to question their own ability.

The Intelligence Testing Movement

Intelligence, that fascinating yet enigmatic "something" that promised to discriminate the able from the less able, defied definition but perhaps could be quantified. With the advent of the 20th century and the influx of immigrants to American shores, there appeared to be a need to devise some means of classifying individuals for education, for work, and ultimately for military service.

Binet and Mental Tests

The story of Alfred Binet (1857–1911) and his search for the meaning and measurement of intelligence has been hailed as a major event in the history of psychology.

Devising such an instrument meant that Binet had to begin with a preconceived notion of intelligence, which he believed consisted of 3 elements:

1. *Mental processes possessing direction*, that is, directed toward the achievement of a particular goal.
2. *The ability to adapt by the use of tentative solutions*, that is, testing the relevance of ideas as one proceeds toward a goal.
3. *The ability to make judgments and to criticize solutions*, that is, objectively evaluating solutions.

When a test item differentiated between normal and subnormal, he retained it; if no discrimination appeared, he rejected it. Binet defined *normality* as the ability to do the things that others of the same age usually do. An American psychologist, Lewis Terman, adapted Binet's work for American usage. Called the *Stanford-Binet*, the test has been repeatedly revised and widely used.

Wechsler's Measures of Intelligence

David Wechsler, a clinical psychologist at New York's Bellevue Hospital, needed a reliable means for identifying the truly subnormal in his examination of criminals, neurotics, and psychotics. Consequently, Wechsler devised a series of tests designed to measure intelligence across the life span.

The adult version is known as the *Wechsler Adult Intelligence Scale–Revised*, and consists of 11 subtests, 6 comprising the verbal scale and 5 forming the performance scale. Consequently, there are 3 possible intelligence scores: *verbal, performance,* and *total IQ.* Many clinicians have found the separation into verbal and performance assessments to be particularly valuable for diagnostic purposes.

Crystallized and Fluid Intelligence

Psychologists have long been intrigued by the notion of *crystallized* and *fluid* intelligence. Crystallized intelligence includes individual differences associated with family, school, and environmental opportunity. Thus, crystallized intelligence is directed at the acquisition of factual knowledge, accumulated information, and basic skills. Fluid intelligence, on the other hand, is active in problem solving and creative efforts, a more flexible and insightful tool than crystallized intelligence.

Research indicates that crystallized intelligence continues to increase into late adulthood, while fluid intelligence begins to decline during the early adulthood years. In the Seattle Longitudinal Study, begun in 1956, Schaie (1994) studied 500 subjects, 25 men and 25 women in each 5-year age bracket from ages 20 to 70. By 1994, about 5,000 individuals had participated in this research. One positive finding has been to show that there is no cognitive collapse throughout the adult years. Most healthy adults begin to demonstrate some decline in fluid intelligence during their 60s and 70s, while crystallized intelligence either remains stable or actually increases until well into the 70s.

Even with this overall pattern, individual variation is typical. For example, some subjects showed a decline as early as their 30s, while others remained mentally alert through their 70s. Summarizing then, cognitive ability holds up well during middle adulthood.

Implications for Health Care Providers

As the middle years progress, the accumulated consequences of an individual's bodily constitution, the environmental forces that have been active over the years, and personality factors such as a positive or negative outlook on life are potent forces in shaping cognitive functioning during these years. Absence of major diseases, a contented family life, and job satisfaction contribute to a stable, or enhanced, mental life. People in their middle years are also concerned about the younger generation and often assume a mentoring role with their own children and younger colleagues. In your work with middle-age adults in clinic, hospital, or business settings, look for signs that suggest tension or stress in their lives.

72 Middle Adulthood: Psychosocial Development

A The Five-Factor Model of Personality

N — Neuroticism (individuals who display considerable anxiety, hostility, depression)

E — Extraversion (individuals who tend to be warm, positively assertive, active)

O — Openness to experience (individuals who tend to be imaginative, creative, open to new ideas)

A — Agreeableness (individuals who are trusting, modest, altruistic)

C — Conscientiousness (individuals who are competent, self-disciplined, achieving)

B Sources of self-efficacy

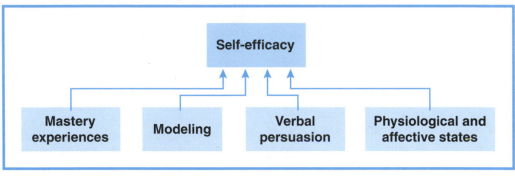

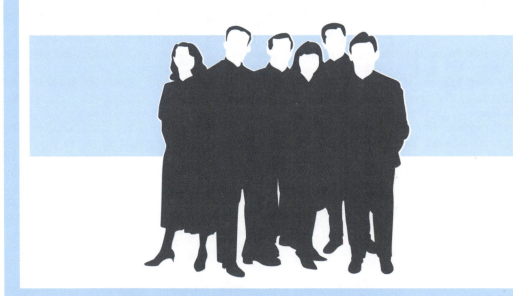

Census figures show that in the decade 1990–2000, an average of 12,000 people per day turned 40. Women between 45 and 54 years make up the fastest-growing age group in the country. Only 10% of Americans over 65 years old have a health problem that prevents them from major activity. These figures testify to a remarkable and influential segment of the population.

Given today's concerns and safeguards about health—diet, exercise, sleep—it comes as no surprise that healthy 50-year-old women will live into their 90s and that healthy males who reach age 65 will survive into their 90s. Longitudinal studies of this age group consistently reveal that both men and women report that they feel at least 10 years younger than their actual age.

Psychologically, Erik Erikson identified the major task of middle adulthood as achieving generativity and avoiding stagnation. *Generativity* refers to a concern for guiding the next generation, the appearance of a sense of caring for the future of family, community, and country. It brings with it greater emphasis on the welfare of children and the assumption of more community and social responsibility.

During these years, the careers of most men will peak: They may be forced into early retirement by a trend toward downsizing; they may shift jobs for a variety of reasons; they may possibly change their career paths. For example, those who have chosen careers requiring great strength, speed, or unusual motor coordination (such as professional athletes, dancers, pilots, etc.) must face the reality of a career change. Many women reenter the work force after an absence of many years as homemakers. Frequently, these women are not overly concerned with money or prestige, but by a desire to work effectively with other adults after spending years with children.

Cohort Differences or Universal Models?

Given these doubts, recent studies have focused on the stability of an individual's personality over the life span. For example, studies such as those by Costa and McCrae (1991, 1994) questioned widely accepted beliefs about middle adulthood, such as the inevitable "midlife crisis." Research has shown that personality remains remarkably stable during these years. The work of Costa and McCrae and others indicates that 5 traits appear with sufficient regularity to create a 5-factor model of personality (Costa and McCrae, 1991, p. 171) (see **Part A**). These 5 factors are consistently found in children, college students, and adults, and in both males and females.

Trait theorists believe there is considerable continuity in these characteristics throughout the lifetime. Such experiences as menopause or retirement *do not* alter the basic personality of most people. Although an individual's personality as a whole remains stable over the years, changes, even dramatic changes, may occur. Physical illness, psychiatric disorder, or catastrophic trauma can radically alter a person's personality.

The Midlife Crisis

Most psychologists today question the inevitability of a midlife crisis. Age alone does not mean that some predetermined crisis looms ahead. There are stresses and strains common to these years, as is true of any age in human development.

In one of their studies, Costa and McCrae (1994) specifically studied the concept of a midlife crisis. They devised a midlife crisis scale that analyzed inner turmoil, marital or job dissatisfaction, and a feeling of declining power. They then used this scale with 500 men ranging in age from 35 to 50. They found that there was no one age at which the scores were significantly higher than at other ages (a conclusion duplicated in many other studies).

Self-efficacy at Midlife

Stanford psychologist Albert Bandura developed the concept of self-efficacy as an insightful tool in understanding people's reactions to life's events. Unless individuals believe they can produce desired results by their actions, they have little incentive to act. Self-efficacy, then, is an excellent tool to explore an individual's reactions to the events of middle adulthood. (**Part B** illustrates the sources of self-efficacy.)

By midlife, most adults have a realistic sense of efficacy in the activities they feel are important. As Bandura (1997, p. 196) noted, a popular myth portrays midlife as a time when personal growth has peaked, youthful goals are abandoned, and efforts to adjust to a static life inevitably lead to an emotional crisis. Quite the reverse is true. The stability and control that maturity has brought to the lives of most people result in time and opportunity to explore new fields, leading to expanded feelings of self-efficacy. Life is never static.

Implications for Health Care Providers

Working in a variety of settings—occupational clinics, outpatient clinics, health club settings—you are in an excellent position to help middle-age adults maintain the quality of their lives by calling attention to risk factors (e.g., safety at work) and measures that promote health, ranging from individual to group counseling. Topics such as methods and diet to reduce heart attacks and strokes, and awareness of the signs of cancer and diabetes should be priorities.

73 Later Adulthood: Physical Health

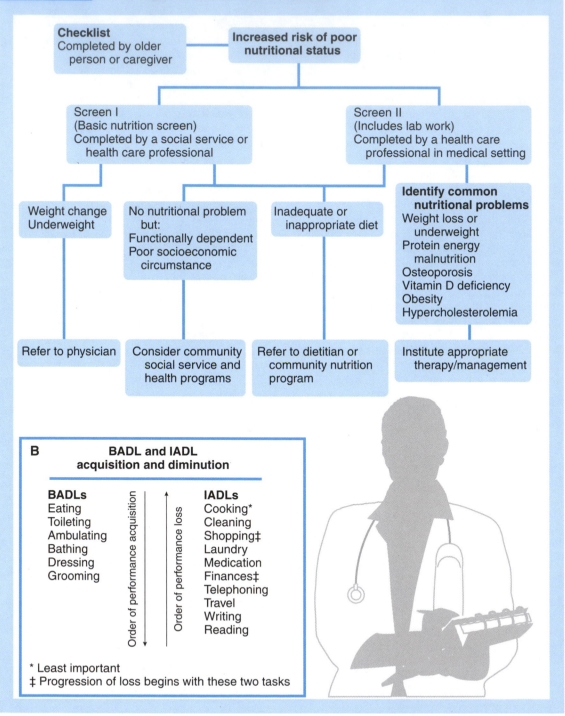

Checklist
Completed by older person or caregiver

Increased risk of poor nutritional status

Screen I
(Basic nutrition screen)
Completed by a social service or health care professional

Screen II
(Includes lab work)
Completed by a health care professional in medical setting

Weight change
Underweight

No nutritional problem but:
Functionally dependent
Poor socioeconomic circumstance

Inadequate or inappropriate diet

Identify common nutritional problems
Weight loss or underweight
Protein energy malnutrition
Osteoporosis
Vitamin D deficiency
Obesity
Hypercholesterolemia

Refer to physician

Consider community social service and health programs

Refer to dietitian or community nutrition program

Institute appropriate therapy/management

B   **BADL and IADL acquisition and diminution**

BADLs
Eating
Toileting
Ambulating
Bathing
Dressing
Grooming

Order of performance acquisition

Order of performance loss

IADLs
Cooking*
Cleaning
Shopping‡
Laundry
Medication
Finances‡
Telephoning
Travel
Writing
Reading

* Least important
‡ Progression of loss begins with these two tasks

Physical Characteristics

Body Composition

There is a 46%–60% decrease in lean body mass and loss of body water after age 65. The matrix of collagen and elastin that transports material between cells becomes cross-linked, resulting in a network of inefficient connective tissue. Collagen becomes insoluble and rigid; elastin becomes brittle, less resilient. The rate at which height is lost increases after age 65, owing to a combination of loss of body water and bone mass, weakened muscle groups, and deterioration of spinal disks. On average, 1.2 cm (1.5–3.0 inches) in height is lost over a lifetime, with women losing more than men.

Nutrition and Weight

Elders typically lose weight, in part due to loss of body water, fat, lean muscle mass, and bone mass. Weight loss may also be attributed to health problems, decline in capacity for self-care, loneliness, and poverty. A decrease in food intake, a decrease in water intake due to concerns about urinary frequency, slowing of peristalsis in the gastrointestinal tract, and lack of exercise increase the risk for malnutrition, dehydration, and constipation. Malnourishment increases vulnerability to even minor illness. An assessment of nutritional status is key to promoting good health later in life (see **Part A**).

Skin

Elders replace epidermal cells every 30 days or more, compared to 20 days or less in younger people. Loss of subcutaneous fat and collagen means that the dermis becomes thinner and loses elasticity. Older skin is more easily damaged, and wound healing is 50% slower than in midlife.

Vision and Hearing

A loss of cells along the optic nerve results in a decline in dynamic visual acuity (i.e., the ability to discriminate detail in moving objects). The reaction time of the pupil to changes in light slows, making it harder to negotiate the dark. Cataracts develop when the lens of the eye becomes more opaque due to oxidative damage to the protein in the lens, a process hastened by exposure to sun.

Atrophy of the ear canal, degenerative changes in the bones of the middle ear, and thickening of the eardrum contribute to hearing loss. The ability to detect higher frequencies (consonant sounds) first diminishes in midlife, followed later by loss in lower frequencies (vowel sounds), decreased ability to hear loud sounds, and difficulties locating the origin of a sound.

Musculoskeletal Changes

Osteoporosis is a decrease in the amount and quality of bone; the remaining bone is normal. Throughout life, bone is constantly being absorbed and rebuilt. With advanced age, more bone is reabsorbed than replaced. As the bone thins, it becomes porous, increasing the risk for fractures. White women with small bone structure are at greatest risk; 15% will fracture a hip. The clinical causes of osteoporosis are related to decreased utilization of calcium in replacing bone, possibly related to estrogen deficiency. Bone density is maintained in women who undergo ERT.

Cardiovascular Changes

The heart muscles become less elastic, and the valves thick and rigid because of infiltration by connective and fibrotic tissue. Contraction time is prolonged; the resting heart rate slows. Oxygen exchange is also less efficient, and aortic volume and systolic blood pressure may rise to compensate. By age 60, the coronary arteries provide 35% less blood to the heart muscle. Half the people over age 60 have narrowing of the coronary arteries as the arterial walls thicken with connective tissue and fatty deposits; half do not. Of those who do, half will develop coronary artery disease.

These changes are most noticeable with exertion or stress. It takes longer for the heart to accelerate to meet the demand for increased blood flow and oxygenation. There is also a slower return to a resting heart rate when the demand ceases. The expected increase in heart rate in response to pain or anxiety may not be manifested as readily in elders due to the slower response time.

Genitourinary Changes

There is a 50% reduction in the kidneys' rate of filtration, causing delays in the clearance of medications and glucose. At the same time, bladder capacity decreases, leading to urinary frequency. Older women may experience stress incontinence when they cough, but incontinence is not a normal part of aging and can be treated. Men continue to produce sperm well into old age, although the testes become smaller. A decrease in the production and concentration of testosterone results in a reduced sperm count and enlargement of the prostate gland. The enlarged prostate blocks the flow of urine, and men experience urinary frequency.

Functional Assessment

A functional assessment is a systematic evaluation of bodily activities of daily living (BADLs) and independent activities of daily living (IADLs) (see **Part B**). A careful assessment can reveal manifestations of disease, open a dialogue on one's living arrangements, and help set realistic goals for living life—not despite infirmity but with it.

In **Part B**, the BADLs are listed vertically in order of acquisition (e.g., eating is mastered before self-bathing). Loss of ability occurs in reverse order, and a person can perform activities above but not below their present level of ability. Attention to grooming typically fails before the ability to get dressed. Among IADLs, loss of ability often begins with managing finances. Individuals can usually perform activities below but not above their current level of competence.

74 Later Adulthood: Cognition

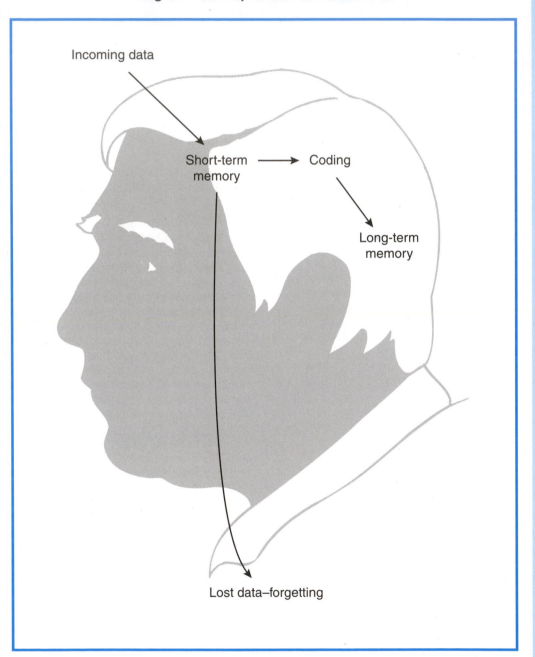

Cognitive development in later adulthood

Incoming data

Short-term memory → Coding

Long-term memory

Lost data–forgetting

Today, people who reach the age of 65 have a good chance of surviving into their 80s, with a 25% chance of making it to 90. But it is the quality of these years that concerns most individuals as they approach later adulthood. Horror stories abound about the decline of cognitive abilities during the 60s, 70s, and 80s (even 90s), but fortunately recent studies (such as the Seattle Longitudinal Study) paint a more promising picture. They clearly show that individuals who maintain their levels of cognitive functioning continue to engage in mental activities, whether it is careful reading of newspapers, doing crossword puzzles, or facing new challenges (such as learning to use a computer).

Cognitive Change: Fact or Fiction?

Research suggests that as people enter these years, their physical stamina, memory, and cognitive processing do not decline as much as previously thought (for an example of this research, see Schaie, 1994). Although some aspects of cognitive functioning (e.g., speed of processing) lose a degree of efficiency, such losses in a healthy 60-, 70-, or 80-year-old are more than offset by gains in knowledge and skill due to experience.

Analysis of the cause of an apparent decline in intelligence (as measured by intelligence tests) leads to several conclusions:

- When **physical health** remains good, cognitive performance suffers only a slight decline.
- **Speed of response** is the time taken to perform any task that involves the CNS such as perception, memory reasoning, and motor movement. It is the basis for efficient cognitive functioning, especially memory (Birren and Fisher, 1992).
- **Attitude,** especially in a testing situation, affects cognitive performance. Test anxiety lowers test scores when older adults find themselves in strange settings.

In assessing levels of intelligence, remember that cognitive functioning encompasses many components: sensory discrimination; attention; perceptual acuity; memory; extent of knowledge; speed of processing, integrating, and synthesizing facts; and the ability to recognize and attack problems. Cognitive performance consists of both gain and loss. For example, reasoning, problem solving, and wisdom hold up well with age and may even improve. Speed of response and memory may show signs of slippage.

To summarize what seems to be happening cognitively during these years, let us again turn to the Seattle Longitudinal Study, remembering the distinctions between fluid and crystallized intelligence (see Chapter 67). Tests of crystallized intelligence (recognizing and understanding words, using numbers, retrieving words from long-term memory) indicate that older adults retain the meaning of words, can still apply numbers, and maintain stable levels of word fluency. Tests of fluid intelligence (identifying principles and rules, rotating objects mentally) show greater decline.

Changes in Memory in the Later Years

Psychologists today believe that memory, rather than being a single component of mind, is made up of different systems and processes. Each system relates to different neuronal networks that play a specialized role in remembering (Schacter, 1996, p. 6).

Consequently, there are various types of memories:

- **Short-term memory** enables brief retention of facts and information because of a system called *working memory* (Schacter, 1996, p. 43).
- **Long-term memory** enables storage of information indefinitely. The significance of long-term memory lies in its survival and adaptation value; humans require an enormous amount of information to survive in a modern society.

Analyzing memory as a network of systems and as a key element in the intelligence of elders leads to an inescapable conclusion: The memories of older adults vary in different situations, ranging from improved performance in some fields, consistent performance in others, and a noticeable decline in still others. For example, after memorizing a list of familiar words, older adults (given no clues) have difficulty remembering them (free recall), but when shown a list of many words, they can identify which were on the original list (recognition) as well as college students can.

Summarizing these studies, Schacter (1996, p. 294) noted that as humans age, the richness of memories for what happened last week or month declines. Older adults remember fewer details of their most recent experiences and rely more on general feelings of familiarity.

Implications for Health Care Providers

Recent findings presented in this chapter suggest that mental decline is not as pronounced in the elderly as was once thought. In fact, many of the elderly have maintained a high level of cognitive ability. Remember, however, that certain aspects of cognitive functioning, such as speed of processing information, show inevitable loss. If you are instructing the elderly in the use of medication, for example, be sure to give them sufficient time to understand your meaning. Consequently, in your contacts with older individuals, encourage them to read, keep in contact with others, and take seminars or classes if they are able. Your goal should be to urge them to keep their minds as active as possible.

75 Later Adulthood: Psychosocial Development—Part A

Psychosocial development in later adulthood

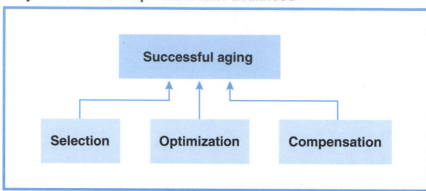

Successful aging

Selection — Optimization — Compensation

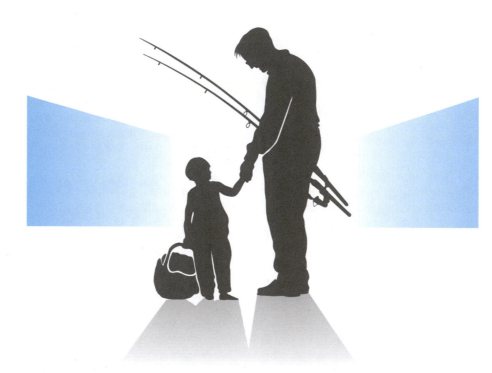

The later years constitute Erikson's final stage of the life cycle: ego integrity versus despair. As Erikson stated (1950, p. 231), those who have taken care of people and things and have adapted to the joys and disappointments that accompany living can harvest the fruits of their lives. Lacking such adjustment leads to feelings of despair because little time remains to search for alternative life choices and also leads to heightened fears of death. Individuals struggle to evaluate and give meaning to all that has occurred: Is there a meaningful pattern and satisfaction in a job well done, or a sense of despair that life should have been lived differently?

To understand how older people feel about their lives, Fisher (1993) interviewed 74 people aged 60 or older. As a result, he divided these years into 5 separate periods:

1. **Continuity with middle age.** Many of the elders interviewed did not feel any abrupt change with old age and retirement, but felt a sense of continuity with their behaviors and activities of middle adulthood. Fisher believed that the added time they could devote to leisure activities substituted for work activities.
2. **Early transition.** Awareness of change or transitions come with the death of a spouse or a serious health problem. Such an abrupt shift made Fisher's subjects aware of the break with middle adulthood and the onset of old age, which occasionally led to feelings of loss and sadness.
3. **Revised lifestyle.** The transitions of the second period frequently required a change in lifestyle, such as a new residence if living alone or reduced activities if illness strikes.
4. **Later transition.** In Fisher's study, many of the older adults had serious illnesses that dictated reduced mobility and loss of independence. Several of his subjects were forced to move in with their children or into retirement communities.
5. **Final period.** Individuals in this phase had to adjust to the circumstances in the fourth period and set new, realistic goals. Most of his subjects faced up to the challenges, but also recognized the inevitability of decline and death.

Successful Aging

If we turn to the positive features of aging—expertise, wisdom, generativity, experience, and so on—we see characteristics that most older adults strive to attain. But are these positive markers the natural result of aging, or are they the benefits of a lifetime of conscious decision making and planned effort? Again, as we have seen so frequently, how individuals interpret the personal experiences of their lives leads to feelings of sadness or despair or a sense of satisfied culmination.

Paul Baltes and colleagues (1992) identified 3 strategies that help older adults in their quest for successful aging: *selection*, *optimization*, and *compensation* (see **Part A**). The first component, *selection*, reflects the reduced capacity every older adult experiences. *Optimization* refers to the ability to preserve a high level of performance by continued effort and added experience. *Compensation* reflects an adjustment in performance when tasks demand a level of response that taxes a person's capacity. Illness, which can be a frequent companion during these years, frequently increases the need for compensation.

Using a television interview with pianist Arthur Rubinstein when he was in his 80s, Baltes and colleagues illustrated how selection, optimization, and compensation interact. Rubinstein described how he maintained a frantic schedule and superb performance as an older adult. First, he reduced the number of pieces he played, an example of selection. Next, he practiced more than he did as a younger man, an example of optimization. Finally, he devised new playing techniques such as slowing down before fast passages to emphasize the change in pace, an example of compensation.

76 Later Adulthood: Psychosocial Development—Part B

Stage	Meaning
Denial	People refuse to believe they are terminally ill, especially when they still feel well.
Anger	People become angry at the "injustice of it all".
Bargaining	Accepting the truth of the diagnosis, people try to "make a deal". "If I do everything you tell me, can I get another year?"
Depression	When nothing works, feelings of futility set in.
Acceptance	Just before death, people usually accept the inevitable.

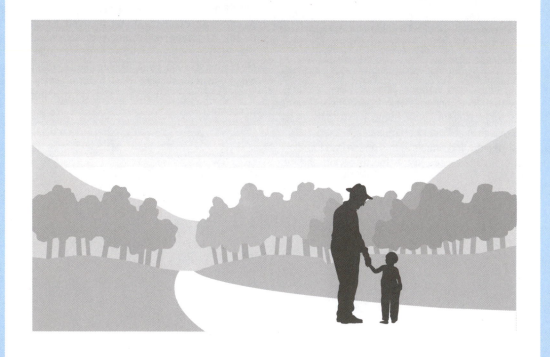

Death and Dying

The later years, however, are associated with thoughts of looming death. The realization of death affects different people in different ways. Some individuals face the reality of death calmly and with careful preparation. They have drawn wills, disposed of assets, and solidified relationships. Others resist any thoughts about dying and grimly struggle to ignore what fate has foreordained. Still others succumb to thoughts of death by retreating into depression. As you can imagine, no matter how prepared a person seems to be for the end, death anxieties creep in. How these are handled and evaluated goes far in determining if one passes through these years in a state of integrity or despair.

Whether one agrees with Elizabeth Kubler-Ross's views on death (1969) or not, she is widely credited for her efforts to call attention to the psychological needs of the dying. Interviewing 200 terminally ill patients, she identified 5 stages that people pass through when they realize that death is inescapable (see **Part A**).

Kubler-Ross herself retreated from the rigidity of a stage theory of death. People simply do not follow a set formula in how they face death. In death as in life, individual differences are the norm. Dying people exhibit many of these characteristics, but they do not unfailingly follow this prescribed pattern. People, as they did in their lives, use individual techniques of coping with death. Also, different cultures place different interpretations on death. Some Native Americans, for example, are taught that since death is part of nature's cycle, it is not to be feared but faced with stoicism and composure. Still, to Kubler-Ross's credit, she has created a sense of awareness and sensitivity to the feelings and emotions of those facing death.

Adapting to Death

Rather than searching for universal patterns of coping with the prospect of death, many researchers have turned to an individual's circumstances as death approaches. In 1 study, 62 women with breast cancer were interviewed 3 months after the diagnosis and their reactions were classified into 5 groups: denial, fighting spirit (optimistic attitudes, seeing the disease as a challenge), stoic acceptance (fatalistic attitude), helplessness/hopelessness, and anxious preoccupation (everything is pessimistic). The survival rate for the different groups is fascinating. After 15 years, only 35% of those whose initial response was denial or fight had died, compared with 76% of the patients in the other categories (Greer, 1991). Since all of the subjects in this study had been in the initial stages of their disease and treatment, the results testify to the powerful impact of psychological processes on disease management.

Where Does Death Occur?

In the United States, about 80% of all deaths occur in hospitals, although the figures are constantly shifting. As more and more people live significantly longer lives, nursing home placement has grown rapidly. These latter years bring serious illness and an inability to receive proper care in the home. The advantages and disadvantages of the terminally ill person remaining at home must be weighed carefully.

Hospice Care

Hospice has done much to make home care of the terminally ill person more acceptable. With its goal of providing appropriate care in a homelike atmosphere, with its emphasis on meeting the range of a patient's needs, and with its recognition of the importance of a dignified death, hospice care has become more appealing as people become familiar with its programs and goals.

Four characteristics have become the hallmark of a hospice program (Wentzel, 1981):

1. Control of chronic pain, which consists of 4 essential parts: the right analgesic agent, in the least amount necessary, at the right time, and in the most effective manner.
2. Realism about death, which includes strong psychosocial support for the patient and family, coupled with realism and truthfulness.
3. The family as the primary unit of caring, which means a recognition that death is usually a social phenomenon; that is, the family context must be considered.
4. Staff support systems, implying that professionalism is compatible with compassion.

Implications for Health Care Providers

Since one of the fastest age groups in the country is older-than-85, category, different perspectives about aging have appeared. Although many positive features of successful aging are now recognized, inevitable physical, cognitive, and psychosocial changes occur. Increasing bouts with illness are common and health maintenance becomes central to the quality of one's lifestyle.

In working with older adults, be alert to any nutritional deficiencies, sleep problems, and lack of physical activity. Adjust your recommendations to the health and vigor of your clients. It is important to encourage their feelings of independence (and urge their family members to do likewise) so that they maintain a positive self-concept. Probably the most important consideration to remember is that these clients need as much psychological support as you can provide to help them adjust to declining functions and impending death.

Directions: For each of the following questions, choose the **one best** answer.

1. Which of the following is an example of health promotion in early adulthood?

(A) Self-breast examinations for women

(B) Stress management

(C) Using seat belts

(D) Being immunized against hepatitis B

2. What is the major reason for obesity during early adulthood?

(A) Maturing of muscles and bones

(B) Overindulgence in food and alcohol

(C) Lack of exercise

(D) Decline in the basal metabolic rate

3. A theorist who analyzed the cognitive workings of early adulthood was

(A) Freud.

(B) Skinner.

(C) Bandura.

(D) Piaget.

4. Schaie believed that young adults differ from adolescents in the way that they _____ their cognitive abilities.

(A) memorize

(B) neglect

(C) analyze

(D) use

5. The early adult years are often referred to as a

(A) time of firsts.

(B) time of crises.

(C) time of anxiety.

(D) time of regression.

6. Famous for his "seasons of life" concept is

(A) Freud.

(B) Maslow.

(C) Levinson.

(D) Valliant.

7. Which of the following is an example of the nonstochastic theory of aging?

(A) Exposure to radiation that causes mutation in DNA

(B) Damage to cell membranes by free radicals

(C) Genetically programmed changes, e.g., menopause

(D) Increase in connective tissue

8. Which of the following is (are) the most significant risk factor(s) for cardiovascular disease?

(A) Smoking and hypertension

(B) Diabetes and high cholesterol

(C) Obesity and stress

(D) Being male

9. The person most responsible for the intelligence testing movement was

(A) Thorndike.

(B) Webster.

(C) Rorschach.

(D) Binet.

10. _____ intelligence tends to be more creative in nature.

(A) Fluid

(B) Crystallized

(C) Convergent

(D) Conceptual

11. Long thought to be inescapable during middle adulthood is

(A) marriage.

(B) divorce.

(C) midlife crisis.

(D) health problems.

12. When people believe they possess the competence to do what needs to be done, they have a sense of

(A) confidence.

(B) self-fulfilling prophecy.

(C) self-expectation.

(D) self-efficacy.

13. What causes osteoporosis?

(A) Decrease in calcium in the diet

(B) Decreased utilization of calcium

(C) History of bone fractures

(D) Small bone structure

14. Which of the following is evidence of heart disease later in life?

(A) Prolonged contraction time of the heart muscle

(B) Increased rigidity of the heart valves

(C) Neither

(D) Both

15. A cognitive ability that seems to decline with age is

(A) assimilation.

(B) speed of processing.

(C) notational accommodation.

(D) schema structuring.

16. Any loss in cognitive functioning in these years may be offset by acquired _____ and _____.

(A) assimilation, accommodation

(B) cognitive, emotional

(C) introjection, regression

(D) knowledge, skill

17. These later years are Erikson's time of integrity or

(A) despair.

(B) transition.

(C) displacement.

(D) rationalization.

18. Widely credited with making the needs of the dying more well known is

(A) Skinner.

(B) Piaget.

(C) Freud.

(D) Kubler-Ross.

PART VII: ANSWERS AND EXPLANATIONS

1. The answer is B.

Primary prevention refers to efforts to prevent disease and injury in healthy people. Examples include immunizations, use of seat belts, and self-breast examinations. Health promotion is directed at increasing one's well-being, in part through healthy lifestyle choices, such as low-fat diet, regular exercise, and stress management.

2. The answer is B.

A weight gain of 10–15 lb between ages 18 and 30 is largely due to the maturing of muscles, bones, and internal organs and an increase in fatty tissue. Overindulgence in food and alcohol, and not a decline in the basal metabolic rate, is the major reason for obesity during this period.

3. The answer is D.

Piaget's analysis of cognitive development has shed light on cognition at all ages. In early adulthood, for example, the characteristics of formal operational thinking help to explain the thought processes of these years.

4. The answer is D.

Faced with more complex problems, young adults tend to apply their knowledge and cognitive abilities more than adolescents do.

5. The answer is A.

So many "firsts" occur during these years (marriage, children, jobs) that this label is a natural.

6. The answer is C.

Attempting to devise a technique that would encompass the varied happenings of the life span, Levinson turned to phases that he could identify because of the pattern or structure that characterized the various ages.

7. The answer is C.

Stochastic theories propose that aging events are random, cumulative, and microscopic. For example, random exposure to radiation can cause mutations in DNA, causing cells to malfunction. The slow accumulation of damage to cell membranes by free radicals (the by-products of oxygen metabolism) is another stochastic theory. The connective tissue theory proposes that chemical reactions bind molecular structures that work best when separate, such as proteins, nucleic acid, and collagen. Nonstochastic theories propose that aging is genetically programmed into the lives of cells. For example, a genetic timetable shuts down the ovaries, causing menopause.

8. The answer is A.

Smoking, hypertension (blood pressure > 160/90 mm Hg), and type I diabetes are the 3 top risk factors for cardiovascular disease (CVD). High cholesterol, obesity, stress, and overuse of alcohol are secondary risk factors. Men and women are at equal risk for CVD. However, men develop the disease almost 10 years earlier than women, and the manifestation of CVD in men and women is different.

9. The answer is D.

Binet's ideas became the foundation for the acceptance and rapid growth of the intelligence testing movement. Unfortunately, Binet's ideas were misinterpreted and produced much of the mischief we have seen in the past several decades.

10. The answer is A.

Fluid intelligence is what humans use when faced with problems. In a highly technological society, fluid intelligence is much needed.

11. The answer is C.

Today, considerable skepticism greets the idea of an inevitable midlife crisis. While crises occur during these years, they result from typical causes—health problems, stress in the home, career concerns—causes that appear at any age.

12. The answer is D.

Self-efficacy, that feeling of justified confidence, is important at all ages, but especially these years when responsibilities have greatly increased.

13. The answer is B.

Osteoporosis is a decrease in the amount of bone; the remaining bone is normal. Throughout life, bone is constantly being absorbed and rebuilt. With advanced age, more bone is reabsorbed than replaced. As the bone thins, it also becomes more porous and its internal latticework is lost. Strength is compromised, increasing the risk for fractures. White women with small bone structure are at greatest risk; 15% will fracture a hip. The clinical causes of osteoporosis are thought to be related to decreased utilization of calcium in replacing bone, possibly related to estrogen deficiency.

14. The answer is C.

Normative cardiovascular changes should not be confused with evidence of disease. With time and age, heart muscles become less elastic, and the valves thick and rigid because of infiltration by connective and fibrotic tissue. Contraction time is prolonged; the resting heart rate slows. Oxygen exchange is also less efficient, and aortic volume and systolic blood pressure may rise to compensate. By age 60, the coronary arteries provide 35% less blood to the heart muscle.

15. The answer is B.

Research has shown that when the ability to process information slows, a person's memory is unable to extract as much information as in earlier years when processing was speedier. More information simply drops out.

16. The answer is D.

If a person remains healthy during these years, any cognitive deficits may be tempered by the experiences acquired.

17. The answer is A.

For those who have not adapted to the pain, joys, and reality of life (and death), despair looms large in these years. In a sense, it is a time of reconciliation with one's self.

18. The answer is D.

Kubler-Ross's work, while challenged on a methodological basis, brought to the fore the need to recognize the needs of those facing death.

REFERENCES

introduction

Dacey, J., Travers, J. (1999). Human development across the lifespan (4th ed.). New York: McGraw-Hill.

Chapter 4

Wertsch, J., Tulviste, P. (1992). L. S. Vygotsky and contemporary developmental psychology. Dev Psychol 28:548–557.
Vygotsky, L. S. (1978). Mind in society. Cambridge, MA: Harvard University Press.

Chapter 5

Bronfenbrenner, U. (1978). The ecology of human development: Experiments by nature and design. Cambridge, MA: Harvard University Press.

Chapter 6

Maslow, A. (1987). Motivation and personality. (Revised by R. Frager, J. Fadiman, C. McReynolds, and R. Coc.) New York: Harper and Row.

Chapter 7

Bandura, A. (1997). Self-efficacy: the exercise of control. New York: Freeman.

Chapter 8

Bruner, J. (1996). The culture of education. Cambridge, MA: Harvard University Press.
Lerner, R. (1991). Changing organism-context relations as the basic process of development: A developmental contextual perspective. Dev Psychol, 27(1):27–32.

Chapter 9

Baenninger, M., Newcombe, N. (1989). Role of experience in spatial test performance: a meta-analysis. Sex Roles 20:327–343.
Brannon, L. (1996). Gender. Boston, MA: Allyn and Bacon.
Eagly, A., Steggen, V. (1986). Gender and aggressive behavior: a meta-analytic review of the social psychological literature. Psychol Bull 100:309–330.
Friedman, L. (1989). Mathematics and the gender gap: a meta-analysis. Rev Educ Res 59:185–213.
Hyde, J., Fennema, E., Lamon, S. (1990). Gender differences in mathematics performance: a meta-analysis. Psychol Bull 107:139–155.
Lips, H. (1997). Sex and gender (3rd ed.). Mountain View, CA: Mayfield.
Maccoby, E., Jacklin, C. (1974). The psychological of sex differences. Stanford, CA: Stanford University Press.

Chapter 10

Betson, D., Michael, M. (1997). Why so many children are poor. Future of Children 72:25–39.
Kozol, J. (1993). Savage inequalities. New York: Crown.

Chapter 15

Marrs, R., Bloch, L., and Silverman, K. (1997). Dr. Richard Marrs' fertility book. New York: Delacorte.

Chapter 20

Brouwers, P., Tudor-Williams, G., DeCarli, C., et al. (1995). Relation between stage of disease and neurobehavioral measures in children with symptomatic HIV disease. AIDS 9:713–720.

Smith, M. L., Minden, D., Netley, C., Read, S. (1997). Longitudinal investigation of neuropsychological functioning in children and adolescents with hemophilia and HIV infection. Dev Neuropsychol 13:69–85.

Chapter 22

Dacey, J., Travers, J. (1999). Human development across the lifespan (4th ed.). New York: McGraw-Hill.

Chapter 23

Ballard, J. L. et al. (1991). New Ballard score, expanded to include extremely premature infants. J Ped 119:417.

Brazelton, Nugent (1995). Neonatal behavioral assessment scale. London: Heinemann.

DeCasper, A., Fifer, W. (1980). Science 208:1174.

Chapter 26

Gibson, E., Walk, R. (1960). The "visual cliff." Sci Am 202:64–72.

Chapter 27

Dacey, J., Travers, J. (1999). Human development across the lifespan (4th ed.). New York: McGraw-Hill.

Springer, S., Deutsch, G. (1998). Left brain/right brain. New York: Freeman.

Temple, C. (1993). The brain. New York: Penguin.

Chapter 28

Baillergeon, R. (1987). Object permanence in 3.5 and 4.5 month old infants. Dev Psychol 23:665–669.

Rovee-Collier, C. K. (1990). The "memory system" of prelinguistic infants. Ann NY Acad Sci 608:517–542.

Chapter 29

Dacey, J., Travers, J. (1999). Human development across the lifespan (4th ed.). New York: McGraw-Hill.

Hulit, L., Howard, M. (1997). Born to talk. Needham, MA: Allyn and Bacon.

Owens, R. (1996). Language development. Needham, MA: Allyn and Bacon.

Pinker, S. (1994). The language instinct. New York: Morrow.

Chapter 30

Brazelton, B., Cramer, B. (1990). The earliest relationship. Reading, MA: Addison-Wesley.

Chess, S., Thomas, A. (1987). Know your child. New York: Basic Books.

Chapter 31

Ainsworth, M. (1973). The development of infant-mother attachment. In B. Caldwell and H. Riccuti (eds.). Review of child development research. Chicago: University of Chicago Press.

Bowlby, J. (1969). Attachment. New York: Basic Books.

Bowlby, J. (1982). Attachment and loss: retrospect and prospect. Am J Orthopsychiatry 52:664–678.

Bowlby, J. (1988). A secure base. New York: Basic Books.

Dacey, J., Travers, J. (1999). Human development across the lifespan (4th ed.). New York: McGraw-Hill.

Main, M. (1996). Introduction to the special section on attachment and psychopathology: overview of the field of attachment. J Consult Clin Psychol 64:237–242.

Chapter 32

Bridges, K. (1932). Emotional development in early infancy. Child Dev 3:324–334.

Goleman, D. (1995). Emotional intelligence. New York: Bantam.

Greenspan, S. (1995). The challenging child. Reading, MA: Addison-Wesley.

Izard, C. (1991). The psychology of emotions. New York: Plenum.

Chapter 33

Capute, A., Accardo, P. (eds.). (1996). Developmental disabilities in infancy and childhood (2nd ed.). Vol. 1: Neurodevelopmental diagnosis and treatment. Baltimore: Paul H. Brookes.

Case, R. (1992). The role of frontal lobes in the regulation of cognitive development. Brain Cognition 20:51–73.

Springer, S., Deutsch, G. (1997). Left brain, right brain: perspective from cognitive neuroscience. New York: Freeman.

Chapter 35

Bibace, R., and Walsh, M. E. (1981). Development of children's concepts of illness. In R. Bibace and M. E. Walsh (eds.). New directions for child development: Children's concepts of health, illness, and bodily functions. San Francisco: Jossey-Bass.

Chapter 36

Bredekamp, S., Copple, C. (eds.). (1997). Developmentally appropriate practice on early childhood programs serving children from birth through age 8. Washington, D.C.: National Association for the Education of Young Children.

Dacey, J., Travers, J. (1999). Human development across the lifespan (4th ed.). New York: McGraw-Hill.

Montessori, M. (1967). The absorbent mind. New York: Dell.

Chapter 37

Dacey, J., Travers, J. (1999). Human development across the lifespan (4th ed.). New York: McGraw-Hill.

Owens, R. (1996). Language development: an introduction. Needham, MA: Allyn and Bacon.

Pinker, S. The language instinct. (1994). New York: Morrow.

Chapter 38

Baumrind, D. (1971). Current patterns of parental authority. Dev Psychol Monogr 4:1–103.

Dunn, J. (1992). Sisters and brothers: current issues in developmental research. In F. Boer and J. Dunn (eds.). Children's sibling relationships. Hillsdale, NJ: Erbaum.

LeVine, R., Miller, P., West, M. (eds.). (1988). Parental behavior in diverse societies. In W. Damon (editor in chief). New directions for child development. No. 40. San Francisco: Jossey-Bass.

Chapter 39

Dacey, J., Travers, J. (1999). Human development across the lifespan (4th ed.). New York: McGraw-Hill.

Vissing, Y. (1996). Out of sight, out of mind. Lexington, KY: University of Kentucky Press.

Walsh, M. (1992). Moving to nowhere. New York: Auburn House.

Chapter 40

Dacey, J., Travers, J. (1999). Human development across the lifespan (4th ed.). New York: McGraw-Hill.

Hetherington, E. M., Stanley-Hagen, M. (1995). Parenting in divorced and remarried families. In M. H. Bornstein (ed.). Children and parenting. Vol. 4. Hillsdale, NJ: Erlbaum.

Wallerstein, J. (1983). Children of divorce: the psychological tasks of the child. Am J Orthopsychiatry 53:230–243.

Wallerstein, J., Blakeslee, S. (1989). Second chances. New York: Ticknor and Fields.

Chapter 41

Clarke-Stewart, A. (1992). Day care (2nd ed.). Cambridge, MA: Harvard University Press.

NICHD (1997). The effects of infant child care on infant-mother attachment security: results of the NICHD study of early child care. Child Dev 68:860–879.

NICHD (in press). Early child care and self-control, compliance and problem behavior at 24 and 36 months. Early Child Care.

Shonkoff, J. (1995). Child care for low-income families. Young Children 50(6):63–65.

Chapter 42

Harter, S. (1990). Issues in the development of the self-concept of children and adolescents. In A. LaGreca (ed.). Through the eyes of a child. Boston, MA: Allyn and Bacon.

James, W. (1890). The principles of psychology. New York: Holt, Rinehart, and Winston.

Lewis, M., Brooks-Gunn, J. (1979). Social cognition and the acquisition of self. New York: Plenum.

Chapter 44

Bem, S. (1985). Androgyny and gender schema theory: a conceptual and empirical integration. In T. B. Sondregger (ed.). Nebraska symposium on motivation: psychology of gender. Lincoln: University of Nebraska Press.

Dabbs, J. M. (1992). Testosterone measurements in social and clinical psychology. J Soc Clin Psychol 11:302–321.

Diamond, M. (1997). Sexual identity and sexual orientation in children with traumatized or ambiguous genitals. J Sex Res 34:199–211.

Money, J., Ehrhardt, A. (1972). Man and woman, boy and girl. Baltimore: Johns Hopkins University Press.

Chapter 45

Berk, L. (1997). Child development (4th ed.). Needham Heights, MA: Allyn & Bacon.

Dacey, J., Travers, J. (1999). Human development across the lifespan (4th ed.). New York: McGraw-Hill.

Garvey, C. (1990). Play. Cambridge, MA: Harvard University Press.

Piaget, J. (1962). Play, dreams, and imitation in childhood. New York: W. W. Norton.

Rybin, K., Fein, G., & Vandenberg, K. (1988). Play. In E. M. Hetherington (ed.). Handbook of child psychology: socialization, personality, and social development (4th ed., pp. 693–744). New York: Wiley.

Chapter 47

Bibace, R., Walsh, M. E. (1981). Development of children's concepts of illness. In R. Bibace and M. E. Walsh (eds.). New directions for child development: children's concepts of health, illness, and bodily functions. San Francisco: Jossey-Bass.

Chapter 48

Dacey, J., Travers, J. (1999). Human development across the lifespan (4th ed.). New York: McGraw-Hill.

Gardner, H. (1983). Frames of mind. New York: Basic.

Gardner, H. (1995). Leading minds. New York: Basic.

Gardner, H. (1997). Multiple intelligences as a partner in school improvement. Educ Leadership 55(1):20–21.

Sternberg, R. (1988). The triarchic mind: a new theory of human intelligence. New York: Viking.

Sternberg, R. (1990). Metaphors of mind: conceptions of the nature of intelligence. New York: Cambridge University Press.

Sternberg, R. (1994). Allowing for thinking styles. Educ Leadership 52(3):36–41.

Sternberg, R. (1996). Successful intelligence. New York: Simon & Schuster.

Chapter 49

Bransford, J., Stein, B. (1993). The IDEAL problem solver. New York: Freeman.

Chapter 50

Gilligan, C. (1977). In a different voice: women's conception of self and of morality. Harvard Educ Rev 47:481–517.

Gilligan, C. (1982). In a different voice. Cambridge, MA: Harvard University Press.

Gilligan, C., Ward, J., Taylor, J. (1988). Mapping the moral domain. Cambridge, MA: Harvard University Press.

Kohlberg, L. (1966). A cognitive-developmental analysis of children's sex-role concepts and attitudes. In E. Maccoby (ed.). The development of sex differences. Stanford, CA: Stanford University Press.

Chapter 51

Hakuta, K., McLaughlin, B. (1996). Bilingualism and second language learning: seven tensions that define the research. In D. Berliner and R. Calfee (eds.). Handbook of educational psychology. New York: Macmillan.

McLaughlin, B. (1990). Development of bilingualism: myth and reality. In A. Barona & E. Garcia (eds.). Children at risk (pp. 65–75). Washington, D.C.: National Association of School Psychologists.

Owens, R. (1996). Language development: an introduction. Needham, MA: Allyn and Bacon.

Reagan, T. (1997). The case for applied linguistics in teacher education. J Teacher Educ 48(3):185–196.

Chapter 52

Greenspan, S. (1993). Playground politics: understanding the emotional life of your school-age child. Reading, MA: Addison-Wesley.

Hartup, W. (1983). Peer relations. In P. Mussen (ed.). Handbook of child psychology. New York: Wiley.

Selman, R., Schultz, L. (1991). Making a friend in youth. Chicago: University of Chicago Press.

Chapter 53

Rutter, M., Maughan, B., Mortimore, P., Ouston, J. (1979). Fifteen thousand hours. Cambridge, MA: Harvard University Press.

Chapter 54

Josephson, M. (1959). Edison. New York: Wiley.

McKim, R. (1972). Experiences in visual thinking. Monterey, CA: Brooks/Cole.

Chapter 55

Dennis, W. (1973). Children of the creche. New York: Appleton-Century-Crofts.

Koluchova, J. (1976). A report on the further development of twins after severe and prolonged deprivation. In A. M. Clarke and A. D. Clarke (eds.). Early experience: myth and evidence. London: Open Books.

Kronenberger, W., Thompson, R. (1990). Dimensions of family functioning in families with chronically ill children: a higher order factor analysis of the Family Environment Scale. J Clin Child Psychol 19(4):380–388.

Rutter, M., Yule, B., Morton, J., Bagley, C. (1975). Attainment and adjustment in two geographical areas. III: Some factors accounting for area differences. Br J Psychiatry 126:520–533.

Werner, E., Smith, R. (1992). Overcoming the odds: high risk children from birth to adulthood. Ithaca: Cornell University Press.

Chapter 56

Capute, A., Accardo, P. (eds.). (1996). Developmental disabilities in infancy and childhood (2nd ed.). Vol. I. Neurodevelopmental diagnosis and treatment. Baltimore: Paul Brookes.

Ireys, H. (1994). Children with special health care needs: evaluating their needs and relevant service structures. Unpublished paper. Institute of Medicine, Johns Hopkins University, Baltimore, MD.

Parker, S., Zuckerman, B. (eds.). (1995). Behavioral and developmental pediatrics: a handbook for primary care. Boston: Little, Brown.

Chapter 57

Tanner, J. M. (1990). Foetus into man. Cambridge, MA: Harvard University Press.

Chapter 58

Allensworth, D., Symons, C., Olds, R. (1994). Healthy Students 2000: an agenda for continuous improvement in America's schools. Kent, OH: American School Health Association.

Centers for Disease Control. (1996). Youth risk behavior surveillance. MMWR 45(SS-4):1–86.

U.S. Department of Health and Human Services. (1990). Healthy People 2000: national health promotion and disease prevention objectives. Washington, D.C.: U.S. Government Printing Office.

Chapter 59

Brooks-Gunn, J., Paikoff, R. (1993). Sex is a gamble, kissing is a game: adolescent sexuality and health promotion. In S. Millstein, A. Petersen, and E. Nightingale (eds.). Promoting the health of adolescents: new directions for the twenty-first century. New York: Oxford University Press.

Centers for Disease Control and Prevention. (1996). Youth risk behavior surveillance 1995: Morbidity and Morality Report Weekly 45(SS-4):1–86.

Dacey, J., Kenny, M. (1997). Adolescent development. Madison, WI: Brown and Benchmark.

Forste, R., Heaton, R. (1988). Initiation of sexual activity among adolescent females. Youth Society 19(3):250–268.

Jones, J., Barlow, D. (1990). Self-reported frequency of sexual urges and fantasies in heterosexual males and females. Arch Sex Behav 19(3):269–279.

Chapter 60

Elkind, D. (1994). Understanding your child. Boston: Allyn and Bacon.

Flavell, F., Miller, P., Miller, S. (1993). Cognitive development. Englewood Cliffs, NJ: Prentice Hall.

Piaget, J., Inhelder, B. (1969). The psychology of the child. New York: Basic Books.

Chapter 61

Elkind, D. (1984). All dressed up and no place to go. Reading, MA: Addison-Wesley.

Fiske, S., Taylor, S. (1984). Social cognition. New York: Random House.

Selman, R., Schultz, L. (1991). Making a friend in youth: developmental theory and pair therapy. Chicago: University of Chicago Press.

Thies, K., Walsh, M. F. (1999). A developmental analysis of cognitive appraisal of stress in children and adolescents with chronic illness. Child Health Care 28(1):15–32.

Chapter 62

Brown, B. (1990). Peer groups and peer cultures. In S. Feldman and G. Elliot (eds.). At the threshold: the developing adolescent. Cambridge, MA: Harvard University Press.

Freud, A., Dann, S. (1951). An experiment in group upbringing. Psychoanal Study of Child 6:127–168.

Lerner, R., Galambos, N. (1998). Adolescent development: challenges and opportunities for research, programs, and policies. In J. Spence, J. Darley, and Donald Foss (eds.). Annual review of psychology. Palo Alto, CA: Annual Reviews.

Selman, R. (1980). The growth of interpersonal understanding: developmental and clinical analysis. New York: Academic Press.

Chapter 63

Marcia, J. (1966). Development and validation of ego identity status. J Pers Soc Psychol 3:551–558.

Marcia, J. (1980). Identity formation in adolescence. In J. Adelson (ed.). Handbook of adolescent psychology. New York: Wiley

Chapter 64

Bandura, A. (1997). Self-efficacy: The exercise of control. New York: Freeman.

Bruner, J. (1966). Studies in cognitive growth. New York: Wiley.

Skinner, B. F. (1971). Beyond freedom and dignity. New York: Knopf.

Weiner, B. (1980). Human motivation. New York: Holt, Rinehart and Winston.

Chapter 65

Bandura, A. (1997). Self-efficacy: The exercise of control. New York: Freeman.

Glueck, S., Glueck, E. (1950). Unraveling juvenile delinquency. Cambridge, MA: Harvard University Press.

Healy, W., Bronner, A. (1936). New light on delinquency and its treatment. New Haven: Yale University Press.

Lerner, R., Galambos, N. (1998). Adolescent development. In J. Spence, J. Darley, and D. Foss (eds.). Annual review of psychology. Palo Alto, CA: Annual Reviews.

Rigoli, R., Hewitt, J. (1991). Delinquency in society. New York: McGraw-Hill.

Travers, J., Elliott, S., Kratochwill, T. (1993). Educational psychology: effective teaching, effective learning. Dubuque, IA: Brown and Benchmark.

Wilson, J., Herrnstein, R. (1985). Crime and human nature. New York: Simon and Schuster.

Chapter 66

Brooks-Gunn, J., Petersen, A. (1991). Studying the emergence of depression and depressive symptoms during adolescence. J Youth Adolesc 20:115–119.

Diagnostic and statistical manual of mental disorders (4th ed.). (1994). Washington, D.C.: American Psychiatric Association.

Wallander, J., Varni, J. (1992). Adjustment in children with chronic physical disorders. In A. LaGreca, L. Siegel, J. Wallander, and C. Walker (eds.). Stress and coping in child health. New York: Guildford Press.

Chapter 67

Belloe, N., Breslow, L. (1972). Relationship of physical health status and health practices. Prev Med 1:409–421.

Pender, N. (1996). Health promotion and nursing practice (3rd ed.). Norwalk, CT: Appleton-Century-Crofts.

Rosenstoch, I. (1974). Historical origin of the health belief model. Health Educ Monogr 2:334.

Chapter 68

Berk, L. (1998). Development through the lifespan. Needham Heights, MA: Allyn and Bacon.

Flavell, J., Miller, P., Miller, S. (1993). Cognitive development. Englewood Cliffs, NJ: Prentice Hall.

Perry, W. (1970). Forms of intellectual and ethical development in the college years. New York: Holt, Rinehart and Winston.

Perry, W. (1981). Cognitive and ethical growth. In A. Chickering (ed.). The modern American college. San Francisco: Jossey-Bass.

Schaie, K. W. (1977). Toward a stage theory of adult cognitive development. Aging Hum Dev 8:129–138.

Schaie, K. W. (1994). The course of adult intellectual development. Am Psychol 49:304–313.

Siegler, R., Richards, D. (1982). The development of intelligence. In R. Sternberg (ed.). Handbook of human intelligence. New York: Cambridge University Press.

Chapter 69

Havighurst, R. (1972). Developmental tasks and education. New York: McKay.

Levinson, D. (1978). The seasons of a man's life. New York: Knopf.

Levinson, D. (1996). The seasons of a woman's life. New York: Knopf.

Valliant, G. (1993). The wisdom of the ego. Cambridge, MA: Harvard University Press.

Chapter 71

Schaie, K. (1994). The course of adult intellectual development. Am Psychol 49:304–313.

Sternberg, R. (1995). Successful intelligence. New York: Simon and Schuster.

Chapter 72

Bandura, A. (1997). Self-efficacy: the exercise of control. New York: Freeman.

Costa, P. T., McCrae, R. (1991). Trait psychology comes of age (pp. 169–204). In T. Sonderegger (ed.). Psychology and aging. Nebraska Symposium on Motivation. Lincoln: University of Nebraska Press.

Costa, P. T., McCrae, R. (1994). Set like plaster? Evidence for the stability of adult personality. In T. F. Heatherton and J. L. Weinberger (eds.). Can personality change? Washing-ton, D.C.: American Psychological Association.

Chapter 74

Baltes, P., Smith, J., Staudinger, U. (1992). Wisdom and successful aging (pp. 123–168). In J. Berman and T. Sonderegger (eds.). Psychology and aging. Nebraska symposium on motivation 1991. Lincoln: University of Nebraska Press.

Bandura, A. (1997). Self-efficacy: the exercise of control. New York: Freeman.

Birren, J., Fisher, L. (1992). Aging and slowing of behavior (pp. 1–38). In J. Berman and T. Sonderegger (eds.). Psychology and aging—Nebraska symposium on motivation 1991. Lincoln: University of Nebraska.

Papalia, D., Olds, S. (1998). Human development. New York: McGraw-Hill.

Schacter, D. (1996). Searching for memory. New York: Basic Books.

Schaie, K. (1994). The course of adult intellectual development. Am Psychol 49(4):304–313.

Chapter 76

Baltes, P., Smith, J., Staudinger, U. (1992). Wisdom and successful aging (pp. 123–168). In T. Sonderegger (ed.). Psychology and aging. Nebraska symposium on motivation. Lincoln: University of Nebraska Press.

Erikson, E. (1950). Childhood and society. New York: W. W. Norton.

Fisher, J. (1993). A framework for describing developmental change among older adults. Adult Educ Q 43:76–89.

Greer, S. (1991). Psychological response to cancer and survival. Psychol Med 21:43–49.

Kubler-Ross, E. (1969). On death and dying. New York: Macmillan.

Thompson, R. (1992). Maturing the study of aging (pp. 245–260). In T. Sonderegger (ed.). Psychology and aging. Nebraska symposium on motivation. Lincoln: University of Nebraska Press.

Wentzel, K. (1981). To those who need it most: hospice means hope. Boston: Charles River Books.

Figure Credits

Chapter 5
Reprinted with permission from Bronfenbrenner, U. (1979). The ecology of human development.

Chapter 8
Table. Data from U.S. Bureau of Census, 1995.

Chapter 9
Parts A–C. Reprinted with permission from Lips, H. (1997). Sex and gender (3rd ed.). Mountain View, CA: Mayfield.
Part D. Based on information from U.S. Department of Justice. (1993). Bureau of Justice statistics sourcebook of criminal justice statistics—1992. Washington, D.C.: U.S. Government Printing Office.

Chapter 10
Part A. Based on U.S. Bureau of Census figures released in September 1997.

Chapter 29
Part A. From Bowlby, J. (1982). Attachment and loss: retrospect and prospect. Am J Orthopsychiatry 52:664–678. Reprinted with permission from the American Journal of Orthopsychiatry. Copyright © 1982 by the American Orthopsychiatry Association, Inc.
Part B. After Dacey, J., Travers, J. (1999). Human development across the lifespan (4th ed.). New York: McGraw-Hill.

Chapter 36
Table. Reprinted with permission from Dacey, J., Travers, J. (1999). Human development across the lifespan (4th ed.). New York: McGraw-Hill.

Chapter 40
Part A. Data from U.S. National Center for Health Statistics, 1997.
Part B. Data from U.S. Bureau of Census, 1997.

Chapter 45
Table. After Berk, 1997; Rubin, Fein, and Vandenberg, 1983; and Dacey, J., Travers, J. (1999). Human development across the lifespan (4th ed.). New York: McGraw-Hill.

Chapter 48
Table. After Gardner, H. (1983). Frames of mind. New York: Basic; Gardner, H. (1995). Leading minds. New York: Basic; Gardner, H. (1997). Multiple intelligences as a partner in school improvement. Educ Leadership 55(1):20–21.

Chapter 50

Table. Based on Kohlberg, L. (1966). A cognitive-developmental analysis of children's sex-role concepts and attitudes. In E. Maccoby (ed.). The development of sex differences. Stanford, CA: Stanford University Press.

Chapter 59

Part A. Centers for Disease Control and Prevention. (1996). Youth risk behavior surveillance 1995: sexual behaviors that contribute to unintended pregnancy and STD. MMWR 45(SS-4):1–86.

Chapter 62

Table. Who's Who Special Report, 1997.

Chapter 66

Part A. Diagnostic and statistical manual of mental disorders (4th ed.). (1994). Washington, D.C.: American Psychiatric Association.

Chapter 68

Table. Siegler, R., Richards, D. (1992). The development of intelligence. In R. Sternberg (ed.). Handbook of human intelligence. New York: Cambridge University Press.

Chapter 70

Part B. Reprinted with permission from Cherry, S. H., Runowicz, C. D. (1994). The menopause book: a guide to health and well-being for women. New York: Macmillan.

Chapter 73

Part A. Courtesy of The Nutrition Screening Initiative, Washington, D.C.

INDEX

Acquired immunodeficiency syndrome (AIDS), 45
Activities of daily living, 183
Adaptation, 7, 137
  resilience and, 135
ADD (attention deficit disorder), 137
Adolescents. *See also* Children.
  body image and, 149
  cognition of, 151, 153
    social, 159
  delinquent, 161
  depression in, 163
  health promotion for, 147
  identity and, 157
  motivation of, 159
  peer relationships of, 155
  pregnant, 149
  puberty and, 3, 145
  sexuality of, 149
  substance use by, 147
  suicide by, 163
Adoption, 51
Adults. *See also* Aging.
  anxieties of, 175
  development of
    cognitive, 173, 179, 185
    psychosocial, 175, 181, 186, 189
  health promotion for, 171, 181
  physical changes of, 177, 183
Adult Attachment Interview, 75
African Americans
  cultural contexts and, 17
  poverty and, 21
Agency, sense of, 103
Aggression
  Bandura on, 15
  control of, 103
  delinquency and, 161
  gender and, 19, 107
  sex and, 3
Aging. *See also* Adults.
  demographics of, 181
  process of, 177, 183
  successful, 187
AIDS, 45
Alcohol use
  by adolescents, 147

birth defects with, 45
  obesity and, 171
  suicide and, 163
Alleles, 29
Androgens, 145
Anger, 77
Antisocial behavior, 161, 163
Anxiety
  adolescent, 155
  adult, 175
  about dying, 189
  Freud on, 3
  homelessness and, 97
  Maslow on, 13
Apgar scores, 59
Appearance-reality problem, 87
Assisted reproductive techniques (ARTs), 37, 51
Asthma, 137
Attachment. *See* Bonding.
Attention deficit disorder (ADD), 137
Attribution theory, 159
Audience, imaginary, 153
Authoritarian parents, 95
Autonomy, 5, 13

Ballard Scale, 59
Bandura, Albert, 15, 159, 181
Behaviorism, 15
  motivation and, 159
Bilingual education, 127
Binet, Alfred, 7, 179
Binocular vision, 65
Biopsychosocial model, 91, 135. *See also* Psychosocial
    development.
Birth defects. *See* Genetic diseases.
Bock, Arlie, 175
Bodily activities of daily living (BADLs), 183
Body mass, 171, 183
Bonding, 49, 75
  day care and, 101
  temperament and, 73
Borderline personality disorder, 163
Brain
  development of, 67, 85
  lateralization of, 67
Brazelton, Berry, 59, 73

Breast-feeding, 63
Bronchopulmonary dysplasia (BPD), 47
Bronfenbrenner, Urie, 11
Bruner, Jerome, 17, 159

Cardiovascular system, 171
  aging of, 177, 183
  childhood, 117
Causality, 87
Cell development, 31
Centration, 87, 119
Chess, Stella, 73
Children. *See also* Infants; Toddlers.
  chronically ill, 137
  creative, 133
  day care for, 101
  delinquent, 135
  depression in, 137
  development of
    cognitive, 119
    language, 127
    moral, 3, 125
    social, 129
  exceptional, 137
  growth of, 117
  homeless, 97
  peer relationships of, 129, 155
  play of, 109, 129
  problem solving by, 123
  resilience of, 135
  siblings of, 95
Chromosomes, 29
  abnormalities of, 41, 43
Chronic illness, 137
Class distinctions, 21
Classification skills, 87, 119
Cocaine
  birth defects with, 45
  suicide and, 163
Cognition. *See also* Social cognition.
  adolescent, 151, 153
  adult, 173, 179, 185
  Bandura on, 15
  brain development and, 67, 85
  childhood, 87, 89, 119
  depression and, 163
  infant, 69
  motivation and, 159
  Piaget on, 7
  Vygotsky on, 9
Collagen, 183
Compulsions, 109
Conception, 31
Concrete operations, 119
Conditioning, operant, 15
Conduct disorders, 163
Conformity, 155
Consciousness, 3, 59
Conservation
  gender and, 105
  perception and, 87, 119
Contextualism, 17
Cramer, Bert, 73

Creativity, 133
Cultural perspectives, 17
  social class and, 21
  Vygotsky on, 9
Cystic fibrosis, 41
Cytomegalovirus (CMV), 45

Dann, Sophie, 155
Day care, 101
Defense mechanisms, 3
Deficiency needs, 13
Delinquency, 135, 161
Deoxyribonucleic acid (DNA), 29
Depression, 77
  adolescent, 163
  childhood, 137
  dying and, 189
  homelessness and, 97
  risks for, 163
Depth perception, 65
Developmental contextualism, 17
Developmental delay, 85, 97, 137. *See also* Mental
    retardation.
Developmentally appropriate practices, 91
Diabetes mellitus, 45, 137
Divorce, 99
DNA (deoxyribonucleic acid), 29
Domestic abuse, 49, 135
Down syndrome, 43, 63
Dream analysis, 3
Drug use, 147, 161
DUPE model, 123
Dying, 189
Dyslexia, 19

Ecology, human, 11
Education. *See also* Learning disabilities.
  bilingual, 127
  creativity and, 133
  early childhood, 91
  homelessness and, 97
  infant, 59, 69
  poverty and, 21
  schools and, 131
  theories of, 15
Effect size, 19
Ego, 3. *See also* Identity; Self.
Egocentric thinking, 153
Elastin, 183
Electra complex, 107
Elkind, D., 151, 153
Embryonic development, 33
Emotional development, 77, 137
Endometriosis, 35
Environmental hazards, 45
Erikson, Erik, 5, 187
  on adolescent identity, 157
  on generativity, 181
  on play, 109
Esteem needs, 13
Estrogen replacement therapy (ERT), 177
Ethics
  development of, 3, 125

of Human Genome Project, 39
   superego and, 3
Ethnicity
   cultural contexts and, 17
   genetic disorders and, 43
Exceptional children, 137
Eye-hand coordination, 85

Fables, personal, 153
Failure to thrive (FTT), 63
Family, 95. *See also* Bonding.
Fear, 77
Feminization of poverty, 21
Fertilization
   in utero, 31
   in vitro, 37
Fetal alcohol syndrome, 45
Fetal development, 33
Follicle-stimulating hormone (FSH), 145
Formal operations, 151, 173
Fragile X syndrome, 43
Fraiberg, Selma, 73
Free association, 3
Freud, Anna, 3, 155
Freud, Sigmund, 3
Friendships, 129

Gardner, Howard, 121
Gender differences, 19
   development of, 105, 107
   flexibility in, 175
   infertility and, 35
   moral development and, 125
   poverty and, 21
   sex-linked disorders and, 41, 43
Generativity, 181
Genetic diseases, 29, 41
   risks for, 43
Genetic traits, 29
Genitourinary system. *See also* Reproductive system.
   aging of, 183
   infertility and, 35
   malformations of, 107
Genotype, 29
German measles, 45
Gestational age, 47
Gifted children, 137
Gilligan, C., 125
Gingivitis, 177
Goleman, Daniel, 77
Gonadotropin-releasing hormone (GnRH), 145
Grasping reflex, 61
Greenspan, Stanley, 77
Growth, 13. *See also* Height.
Guilt, 77
   Erikson on, 5
   Freud on, 3

Hair, 171, 177
Handedness, 85
Hand-eye coordination, 85
Happiness, 77
Head circumference, 49, 63

Health Belief Model, 171
Health promotion
   for adolescents, 147
   for adults, 171, 183
Healthy people 2000, 147
Hearing, 177, 183
Heath, Clark, 175
Height
   adult, 171, 183
   childhood, 117
   infant, 63
   toddler, 85
Hermaphroditism, 107
Hispanics
   cultural contexts and, 17
   poverty and, 21
Hodgkin's disease, 29
Holophrases, 71
Homeless children, 97
Hormones, pubertal, 145
Hospice care, 189
Human ecology, 11
Human Genome Project (HGP), 29, 39
Human immunodeficiency virus (HIV)
   infants and, 45
   sperm banks and, 37
Humanistic psychology, 13
Hydrocephalus
   diabetes and, 45
   ventricular hemorrhage and, 47
Hyperactivity disorder, 137
Hyperglycemia, 45, 137

Id, 3
Identity. *See also* Self.
   adolescent, 157
   adult, 187
   Erikson on, 5, 157, 187
   Freud on, 3
   set, 119
Imaginary audience, 153
Impulse control, 103, 129
   delinquency and, 161
Independence, 5, 13
Independent activities of daily living (IADLs), 183
Individuals with Disabilities Education Act (IDEA), 137
Infants. *See also* Children; Prematurity.
   assessment of, 59
   bonding and, 49, 75
   development of
     brain, 67
     cognitive, 69
     emotional, 77
     language, 71
     motor, 65
     sensory, 65
   growth of, 63, 65
   HIV disease in, 45
   learning by, 59, 69
   memory of, 69
   nutrition of, 63
   reflexes of, 61
   relationships of, 73, 75

Infants (*continued*)
    sleep of, 63
    smiles of, 77
Infectious diseases, 45
Inferiority, 5. *See also* Self.
Infertility
    adoption and, 51
    causes of, 35
    therapy for, 37
Integumentary system, 171
    aging of, 177, 183
Intelligence
    fluid, 179
    gender and, 19
    gifted children and, 137
    tests of, 7, 179
    theories of, 121
    types of, 121
Internalization, 9
Interpersonal intelligence, 121
Interpersonal relationships, 75, 129, 155. *See also* bonding.
Intimacy, 5, 175
Intrauterine devices (IUDs), 35
Izard, Carroll, 77

Jacklin, C., 19
James, William, 103

Kinesthetic intelligence, 121
Klinefelter's syndrome, 43
Kohlberg, Lawrence, 125
Kozol, Jonathan, 21
Kubler-Ross, Elizabeth, 189

Language
    acquisition of, 71, 93
    development of, 127
    gender and, 19
    intelligence and, 121
    proficiency in, 17
    Vygotsky on, 9
Lateralization, brain, 67
Lead poisoning, 45
Learning. *See also* Education.
    creativity and, 133
    infant, 59, 69
    schools and, 131
    theories of, 15
Learning disabilities, 137
    cocaine and, 45
    prematurity and, 47
Lerner, Richard, 17
Leukemia, 45
Levinson, Daniel, 175
Life structure, 175
Love, 13, 77
Low birth weight, 47
Luteinizing hormone (LH), 145

Maccoby, E., 19
Macrosystems, 11
Marcia, J., 157
Marijuana, 147

Maslow, Abraham, 13
Maternal bonding. *See* Bonding.
Mathematics
    gender and, 19
    intelligence and, 121
Meiosis, 31
Memory. *See also* Cognition.
    aging and, 185
    childhood, 89
    infant, 69
Menopause, 177
Mental health problems
    adolescent, 163
    childhood, 137
    homelessness and, 97
Mental retardation, 43, 97, 137
    infectious diseases and, 45
    prematurity and, 47
Microsystems, 11
Midlife crisis, 181
Miscarriage, 43
Mitosis, 31
Montessori, Maria, 91
Moral development, 3, 125. *See also* Ethics.
Moro reflex, 61
Motivation, 159
Motor development
    infant, 65
    toddler, 85
Multiculturalism, 17
    moral development and, 125
    Oedipus complex and, 107
Multiple intelligences, 121
Musculoskeletal system, 171
    aging of, 177, 183
    toddler, 85
Musical intelligence, 121

National Association of Education of Young Children (NAEYC), 91
Needs, hierarchy of, 13
Neonatal assessment, 59
Neurological development, 67
New York Longitudinal Study (NYLS), 73
Nutrition
    adolescent, 147
    aging and, 183
    childhood, 117
    infant, 63

Obesity, 17, 171
    childhood, 117
Object permanence, 69
Oedipus complex, 3, 107
Osteoporosis, 177
Ovum, 31
    donation of, 37
    puberty and, 145

Parenting, 95. *See also* Bonding.
Pavlov, Ivan, 15
Peers
    conformity to, 155

relationships with, 129, 155
Perceptual development, 65
Periodontitis, 177
Permissiveness, 95
Perry, William, 173
Personal fables, 153
Personality, 3. *See also* Identity.
Perspective taking, 153, 155
Phenotype, 29
Phenylketonuria (PKU), 41
Physiological needs, 13
Piaget, Jean, 7
    alternatives to, 89
    concrete operations stage of, 119
    formal operations stage of, 173
    on play, 109
    preoperational stage of, 87
    preschool education and, 91
    sensorimotor stage of, 69
Placenta previa, 45
Play behavior, 109, 129
Pleasure principle, 3
Posttraumatic stress disorder (PTSD), 137
Poverty, 21
Preconscious, 3
Prematurity. *See also* Infants.
    Ballard Scale of, 59
    complications of, 47
    growth patterns of, 49
    head circumference and, 49
    infant growth and, 63
    risks for, 49
    terms for, 47
Prenatal development, 45
Preoperational period, 87
Preschool programs, 91. *See also* Toddlers.
Prestige, 13
Preventricular-intraventricular hemorrhage (PIVH), 47
Problem solving, 123
Proximal development zone, 9
Psychiatric problems. *See* Mental health problems.
Psychoanalysis, 3
Psychosexual development, 3
Psychosocial development, 5. *See also* Biopsychosocial
        model.
    adult, 175, 181, 186, 189
Puberty, 145. *See also* Adolescents.
    body image and, 149
    Freud on, 3
Pulmonary system, 171
Punishment, 15

Radiation exposure, 45
Rape, 149
Reciprocal interactions, 73
Reflexes, 61
Reinforcement, 15
Relationships, 73, 129. *See also* Bonding.
    peer, 129, 155
Reproductive system, 171
    aging of, 177, 183
    infertility and, 35
    malformations of, 107

Resilience, 135
Respiratory distress syndrome (RDS), 47
Retardation. *See* Mental retardation.
Ribonucleic acid (RNA), 29
Rooting reflex, 61
Rubella, 45
Rutter, Michael, 131
Rwanda, 17

Safe sex, 149
Safety
    childhood, 117
    need for, 13
Schaie, K. Warner, 173
Schools. *See also* Education.
    learning and, 131
    poverty and, 21
Seattle Longitudinal Study, 185
Self, 3, 103. *See also* Identity.
Self-actualization, 13
Self-control, 103, 137
Self-efficacy, 159, 181
Self-esteem, 13, 103
Sensorimotor period, 7, 69
Sensory development, 65
Set identity, 119
Sex hormones, 145
Sex-linked disorders, 41, 43
Sexual abuse, 135
Sexuality
    adolescent, 149
    adult, 171, 175
Sexually transmitted diseases (STDs)
    adolescents and, 149
    fetal effects of, 45
    sperm banks and, 37
Sexual Maturity Rating Scale, 145
Shame, 77
    Erikson on, 5
    Freud on, 3
Siblings, 95
Sickle-cell anemia, 41
Skin, 171
    aging and, 177, 183
Skinner, B. F., 15
Sleep cycle, 63
Small for gestational age (SGA), 47
Smiles, infant, 77
Smoking
    by adolescents, 147
    fetal effects of, 45
Social and economic status (SES), 11
Social class, 21
Social cognition, 15. *See also* Cognition.
    adolescent, 153, 159
    childhood, 129
Social development, 129
Social schemas, 153
Sociocultural influences, 9, 17
Spatial perception, 69
    gender and, 19
    intelligence and, 121
Sperm, 31

sperm (*continued*)
  donation of, 37
  infertility and, 35
  puberty and, 145
Spina bifida, 41
Stanford-Binet test, 179
Stereotyping, gender, 19
Sternberg, Robert, 121
STORCH syndrome, 45
Strange situation technique, 75, 101
Stress, resilience to, 135
Substance abuse, 147, 161
Sucking reflex, 61
Suicide, 163
Superego, 3
Surfactant, 47
Syphilis, 45. *See also* Sexually transmitted diseases.

Tanner, J. M., 145
Tay-Sachs disease, 41
Technology gap, 21
Teeth, 171, 177
  deciduous, 117
Temperament, 73
Teratogens, 45
Terman, Lewis, 179
Testosterone, 145
Thomas, Alexander, 73
Time-outs, 103
Tobacco use
  by adolescents, 147
  fetal effects of, 45
Toddlers. *See also* Children.
  day care for, 101
  development of
    brain, 85

    cognitive, 87, 89
    gender, 105, 107
    social, 95, 101
  education for, 91
  growth of, 85
  language acquisition by, 93
  play of, 109
Toxoplasmosis, 45
Trauma, 135, 137
  childhood, 117
  therapy after, 17
Trisomy 21, 43, 63
Turner's syndrome, 43

Unconscious, 3
Universal constructivism, 7

Valliant, George, 175
Varicocele, 35
Violence. *See* Aggression.
Vision
  aging and, 177, 183
  development of, 65, 85
Vygotsky, Lev, 9, 91

Wallerstein, Judith, 99
Wechsler, David, 179
Weight
  aging and, 171, 177, 183
  childhood, 117
  infant, 63
Work ethic, 11

Zone of proximal development, 9
Zygote, 31

BUILD *Your Library*

This book and many others on numerous different topics are available from SLACK Incorporated. For further information or a copy of our latest catalog, contact us at:

Professional Book Division
SLACK Incorporated
6900 Grove Road
Thorofare, NJ 08086 USA
Telephone: 1-856-848-1000
1-800-257-8290
Fax: 1-856-853-5991
E-mail: orders@slackinc.com
www.slackbooks.com

We accept most major credit cards and checks or money orders in US dollars drawn on a US bank. Most orders are shipped within 72 hours.

Contact us for information on recent releases, forthcoming titles, and bestsellers. If you have a comment about this title or see a need for a new book, direct your correspondence to the Editorial Director at the above address.

Thank you for your interest and we hope you found this work beneficial.